THE SCIENTIFIC BASIS OF PSYCHIATRY

The achievements of modern medicine have been largely derived from the understanding of biological structure and function which has accrued from advances in a number of basic sciences. On the foundations of such well-established fields as anatomy, physiology, pathology, bacteriology, pharmacology, genetics and immunology it has been possible to construct a clinical science directed towards the causation and rational treatment of many physical diseases. The slower development of psychological medicine can be attributed partly to historical factors bearing on its development and status. In addition, however, progress has been retarded by the innate complexity of a subject which one of its most distinguished representatives has defined as 'the study of abnormal behaviour from the medical standpoint'. The study of human behaviour goes beyond structure and function to incorporate the psychological and social sciences, and so calls for a wider range of scientific inquiry than is required for most other branches of medicine. The purpose of this series of monographs is to provide individual accounts of those disciplines which constitute the scientific basis of psychiatry.

Each volume is written by a practising scientist whose work is related to psychiatric practice and theory so that his/her review of a particular subject reflects a personal contribution and outlook. Together they are intended to provide a conspectus on the problems and challenges posed by a major and growing branch of medicine.

Other titles in the Series

D.J. Hand *Artificial Intelligence and Psychiatry*
B.I. Donovan *Hormones and Human Behaviour*

The benzodiazepine receptor:

drug acceptor only or a physiologically relevant part of our central nervous system?

WALTER E. MÜLLER

Psychopharmacological Laboratory, Central Institute of Mental Health, D-6800 Mannheim, FGR
Professor of Pharmacology and Toxicology, Faculty of Clinical Medicine Mannheim, Ruprecht-Karls-University, Heidelberg

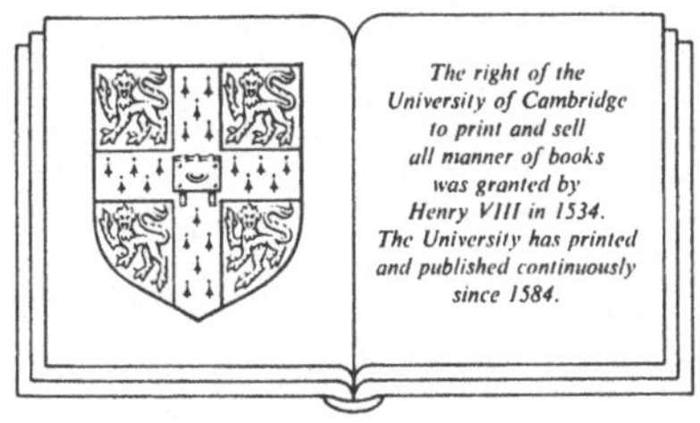
The right of the
University of Cambridge
to print and sell
all manner of books
was granted by
Henry VIII in 1534.
The University has printed
and published continuously
since 1584.

CAMBRIDGE UNIVERSITY PRESS

Cambridge

New York New Rochelle Melbourne Sydney

CAMBRIDGE UNIVERSITY PRESS
Cambridge, New York, Melbourne, Madrid, Cape Town, Singapore, São Paulo, Delhi

Cambridge University Press
The Edinburgh Building, Cambridge CB2 8RU, UK

Published in the United States of America by Cambridge University Press, New York

www.cambridge.org
Information on this title: www.cambridge.org/9780521115278

First published 1987
This digitally printed version 2009

A catalogue record for this publication is available from the British Library

Library of Congress Cataloguing in Publication data

Müller, Walter E. (Walter Erhard), 1947–
The benzodiazepine receptor.

(The Scientific basis of psychiatry; 3)
Bibliography
Includes index.
1. Benzodiazepines – Receptors. 2. Neural
transmission – Regulation. 3. GABA – Physiological
effect. I. Title. II. Series. [NDLM:
1. Benzodiazepines – metabolism. 2. Receptors,
GABA-Benzodiazepines – metabolism. W1 SC836H v.3 /
QV 77.9 M958b]
RM666.B42M85 1987 615′.788 87-787

ISBN 978-0-521-30418-4 hardback
ISBN 978-0-521-11527-8 paperback

CONTENTS

PREFACE

The last 10 years have been very fruitful in elucidating the mechanism of action of the benzodiazepines. Consequently, a clear and definite concept (and not 'just another hypothesis') can presently explain how these important drugs work in our brain. Most of these fascinating new findings are centred on the discovery of a highly specific benzodiazepine binding site in the central nervous system, usually called the 'benzodiazepine receptor'. It is obvious that these new developments are of major interest not only for the basic neuroscientist, but also for the clinician who prescribes benzodiazepines and who wants to know how these drugs work, not only to improve his knowledge of neuropharmacology but also to effect a better and more rational therapeutic use of these drugs.

Since it is the intention of the series '*The scientific basis of psychiatry*' to close the gap between allied basic sciences and research and clinical practice in psychiatry and neurology, the present volume not only gives an overview about the present knowledge on the mechanism of action of the benzodiazepines, but also intends to point specifically to possible implications of these new developments for research and clinical use of these drugs in both clinical disciplines. Accordingly, this is not a book specifically written for the specialist already working in the field of benzodiazepine research. However, some of them might find Chapters 6 (physiological function) and 7 (pathological changes) useful, since these aspects have not been reviewed in such detail before.

As is necessarily the case with every scientific review, a certain selection had to be made. This selection, which reflects my own opinion, concentrates on the well-documented facts concerning basic molecular pharmacological aspects, but it intentionally also covers the putative physiological functions and their possible pathological disturbances –

aspects of direct importance for both clinical disciplines – in a much broader fashion.

Finally, I am obliged to several people for their help and encouragement while I was writing the manuscript. First, to Professor Heinz Häfner, Director of the Central Institute of Mental Health, Mannheim, who suggested that I should write this book and who encouraged me to continue after I had started; secondly, to the publishers, who waited so patiently for the final version; thirdly, to Miss Ingrid Buttler, who typed the manuscript; and last, to my wife, Heidrun, and my children, Helge F., Ulf J. and Juliane K., who tolerated so many hours of my absence from home.

Walter E. Müller

Central Institute of Mental Health, Mannheim
1986

1

Introduction

Andererseits steht zu erwarten – und darin scheint mir ein nicht unerheblicher Nutzen dieser 'Pharmakopsychologie' zu liegen – daß wir bisweilen umgekehrt in die Lage kommen werden, aus der besonderen Wirkung, die ein schon genauer bekanntes Mittel auf einen bestimmten psychischen Vorgang ausübt, die wahre Natur dieses letzteren besser zu erkennen.

On the other hand, and this seems to be a distinct advantage of this 'pharmacopsychology', we might be able to learn from a specific effect of a given drug on a specific psychic symptom something about the true nature of this symptom.

E. Kraepelin (1892)

The hope that knowledge about the exact mechanisms of action of psychotropic drugs will finally lead us to a better understanding about what is wrong in the brains of our psychiatric or neurologic patients is as old as the first experiments in modern psychopharmacology at the beginning of the twentieth century (see above, the quotation of Emil Kraepelin). The concept, advanced nearly 100 years ago, still represents one of the major strategies of recent research in biological psychiatry (Carlsson, 1978). For example, findings about the antidopaminergic activity of neuroleptics and about the effects of antidepressive drugs at noradrenergic and/or serotoninergic synapses have been milestones for the formulation of the dopamine hypothesis of schizophrenia or the amine hypothesis of affective disorders respectively. Yet, as the final biochemical mechanism of action of both classes of drugs is not known, defined biochemical disturbances have not yet been identified in the brains of schizophrenic or depressive patients. Thus, if we consider the enormous amount of basic and clinical research done in this field, we have to realize that, as simple as the concept looks and as valid as it might be, its final results might only be reached after a long and very stony journey. After realizing these difficulties, it seems interesting to ask how much better this concept can be applied to the third major class of therapeutically important psychotropic drugs, the anxiolytics. Anxiolytics – and this means today nearly exclusively benzodiazepines – appear to be particularly interesting. Although very young drugs, benzodiazepines are today the most-prescribed of all psychotropic drugs. Moreover, our knowledge about the mechanism of action is much more advanced in the case of the benzodiazepines than in the case of the neuroleptics or antidepressives. Thus, coming back to Kraepelin's concept again, one feels tempted to speculate that benzodiazepines might represent much better tools for gaining insight into brain function than the two other classes of drugs. Accordingly, it is the major purpose of the present book to see how much this speculation can be substantiated. Since most of the readers will not be familiar with all new aspects of benzodiazepine receptor research, these will be reviewed in the first three chapters. Most of the space, however, will deal with the question of how much the presence of a benzodiazepine-specific receptor improves our knowledge about general aspects of brain function and especially about its pathological disturbances.

1.1 From chlordiazepoxid to the first rank in the list of most frequently prescribed drugs

The first member of the group of benzodiazepines was chlordiazepoxid, synthesized in 1955. Its chemical structure and name are given in Fig. 1.1. Its seven-membered heterocyclic ring, which was a novel chemical structure at this time (see Sternbach, 1973), has subsequently been used to name a steadily growing number of drugs related to this basic chemical structure and with fairly similar pharmacological properties. Chlordiazepoxid was introduced into clinical practice in 1960 and its first congener, diazepam, only 3 years later. Since that time, several thousands of benzodiazepines have been synthesized and tested for activity, and more than 20 have been introduced into clinical use.

One of the most fascinating phenomena related to the benzodiazepines is the rapid acceptance these drugs have found by clinicians as well as by patients. Only 16 years after the introduction of chlordiazepoxid and only 13 years after the introduction of diazepam, diazepam itself ranked second among the most-prescribed drugs in England, only surpassed by paracetamol (Table 1.1). Six benzodiazepines taken together accounted for more than 7% of all prescriptions filled out in England in 1976 (Table 1.1). Similar data have been reported for many other western countries (Blaha & Brückmann, 1983; Müller-Oerlinghausen, 1986). Estimates prepared

Table 1.1 *Prescription frequency in England in 1976*

Prescription frequencies for benzodiazepines in England in 1976 in relation to the total number of prescriptions and to the number of prescriptions filled out for paracetamol (the most frequently prescribed drug in this survey).

Drug	Number of prescriptions	%
Paracetamol	16 161 000	5.5
Diazepam	9 114 000	3.1
Nitrazepam	7 947 000	2.7
Chlordiazepoxid	3 097 000	1.1
Flurazepam	542 000	0.2
Oxazepam	349 000	0.1
Medazepam	276 000	0.1
All benzodiazepines	21 325 000	7.3
All prescriptions	292 638 000	100.0

Source: According to Blaha & Brückmann, 1983.

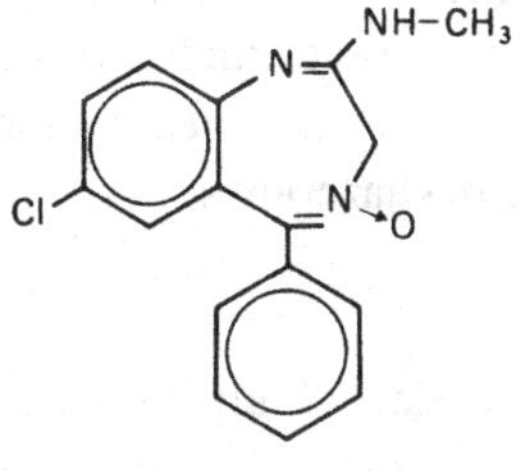

Chlordiazepoxid

(7-chloro-N-methyl-5-phenyl-3H-1,4-benzodiazepin-2-amine-4-oxide)

(IC_{50} = 350)

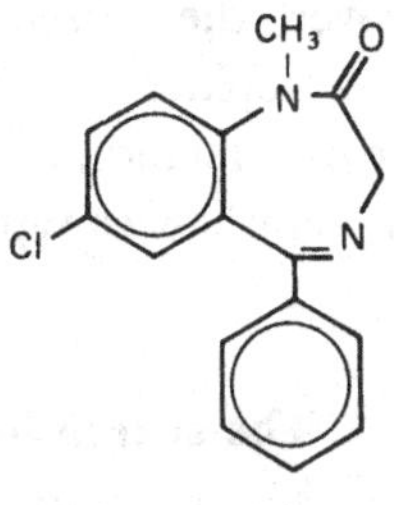

Diazepam

(7-chloro-1,3-dihydro-1-methyl-5-phenyl-2H-1,4-benzodiazepine-2-one)

(IC_{50} = 8)

Fig. 1.1. Structural formulae and chemical names of the two first members of the group of benzodiazepine drugs, chlordiazepoxid and diazepam. IC_{50} indicates the half-maximal inhibitory concentration for *in vitro* benzodiazepine receptor binding (in nmol/l)(as described in detail in § 2.1).

for several European countries suggest that between 10 and 20% of the adult population take a benzodiazepine drug at least once a year, with quite impressive differences between some of the countries (Lader, 1978; Bellantuono *et al.*, 1980; Rickels, 1981; Blaha & Brückmann, 1983; Müller-Oerlinghausen, 1986). It seems highly likely that any use of drugs at such an extent can barely be justified medically. Accordingly, several authors have expressed major concerns about what they call a medical misuse of benzodiazepines (Lader, 1978; Rickels, 1981; Tyrer, 1984; Catalan & Gath, 1985). The concern about the obvious misuse of benzodiazepines has been greatly enhanced by the realization during the last few years that problems of drug dependence occur more frequently than we had thought for many years of clinical use of these drugs (Schöpf, 1983; Tyrer *et al.*, 1983; Ashton, 1984; Tyrer, 1984; Catalan & Gath, 1985). It is not within the scope of this book to discuss further the problems associated with the use and probable misuse of benzodiazepines; these problems have been mentioned mainly to illustrate again the wide acceptance these drugs have found during the last 20 years.

It is obvious that this rapid acceptance by the medical profession would not have taken place if the benzodiazepines were not highly active and also relatively safe drugs, which are used today for a broad spectrum of therapeutic indications, not only in psychiatry and neurology, but also in nearly all medical disciplines (Table 1.2). Since an exact knowledge about the mechanism of action is one of the fundamentals of rational drug therapy, especially if the drugs are as frequently used as the benzodiazepines, to know how benzodiazepines act is important even for their therapeutic use. Moreover, the search for the molecular mechanism of action of the benzodiazepines was always motivated by the hope of finding a key for a better understanding of the biological basis of fear and anxiety and other brain disturbances typically treated with benzodiazepines.

1.2 The search for the mechanism of action, from the very beginning to a specific neuronal receptor

Even the first experiments with chlordiazepoxid demonstrated quite soon that this type of drug exhibits sedative–hypnotic, anxiolytic and anticonvulsive, as well as central muscle-relaxant properties (see Schallek *et al.*, 1979). These four major properties account for all other pharmacological effects of the benzodiazepine in various animal models and for the related therapeutic uses (Table 1.2).

For more than 10 years of extensive use of the benzodiazepines, very little was known about the biological or biochemical basis of their activity. The fourth edition of Goodman & Gilman's standard textbook of pharmacology printed in 1970 stated that 'the effects of this compound [chlordiazepoxid] upon the brain are not well known'. The total discussion about benzodiazepines (all aspects) amounted to only four pages (Table 1.3). Ten years later, in the sixth edition of the same textbook, the total space devoted to benzodiazepines had increased more than fourfold. The reasons for this enormous increase are not only the increasing therapeutic use of these drugs, but also major advances in our understanding of benzodiazepine action. More specifically, two major discoveries were made within the 10 years from 1970 to 1980.

1. Evidence from biochemical, neuropharmacological and electrophysiological experiments indicated that the action of the benzodiazepines at the neuronal level is in some ways linked to that of the major inhibitory neurotransmitter GABA (Costa *et al.*, 1975; Fuxe *et al.*, 1975; Haefely *et al.*, 1975).
2. Specific benzodiazepine binding sites were identified in the mammalian brain, specifically located within GABAergic synapses and acting as the primary target of benzodiazepine drugs (Möhler & Okada, 1977; Squires & Braestrup, 1977).

Table 1.2 *The major pharmacological properties of the benzodiazepines and their corresponding therapeutic uses*

Pharmacological actions	Therapeutic indications
Antipunishment and antifrustration activity, behavioural disinhibition	Anxiety, anxious depression
Arousal reduction, antiaggressive activity	Hyperemotional states
Facilitation of sleep	Insomnia
Anticonvulsant action	Various forms of epileptiform activity
Attenuation of centrally mediated autonomic nervous and endocrine responses to emotions and to excessive afferent stimuli	Psychosomatic disorders (cardiovascular, gastrointestinal, hormonal)
Central muscle relaxation	Somatic and psychogenic muscle spasms, tetanus
Potentiation of the activity of centrally depressant agents, anterograde amnesia	Surgical anaesthesia

Source: According to Haefely *et al.*, 1981.

Both findings have finally led to our present concept of a specific benzodiazepine receptor as a GABA-receptor-regulating subunit of the postsynaptic part of GABAergic synapses (see § 4.2 and 4.3). Thus, our present understanding of the molecular mechanism of action is much better for the benzodiazepines than for the two other important classes of psychotropic drug, the neuroleptics and the antidepressives.

1.3 Drug acceptor or classical receptor? Some semantic and theoretical considerations

If we come back to the major aspect of the present book, the question of how far we can use our advanced knowledge about the mechanism of action of these drugs to get further insight into several aspects of brain function, we soon realize that the main key to this problem is the question about the physiological role of the specific benzodiazepine recognition sites. Since these sites have to be activated by an agonist to function at the neuronal level, the question about the physiological role implies the question about the endogenous agonist acting at these sites. The fact that these sites are now generally termed 'benzodiazepine receptors' (as in the title of this book) does not imply that this question has already been answered. It indicates only our present rather sloppy use of the classical term receptor, which means a more or less specific receptive

Table 1.3 *Benzodiazepines as space in a pharmacology textbook*

The total number of pages covering benzodiazepines in the fourth and sixth editions of Goodman & Gilman's textbook of pharmacology (Goodman & Gilman, 1970 and 1980).

Therapeutic use	Number of pages of discussion	
	Fourth edition (1970)	Sixth edition (1980)
Anxiolytic	3.0	4.0
Anticonvulsive	1.0	2.0
Hypnotic	0.2	10.0
Muscle relaxant	—	0.2
Anaesthetic	—	0.3
Premedication	—	0.2
Total	4.2	16.7

site at a biological macromolecule for an endogenous substance, which by virtue of interacting with the receptor site induces a biological response (Table 1.4). A drug is an agonist if it binds to the receptor and elicits a response similar to that of the endogenous ligand, but it is an antagonist if it binds to the receptor without eliciting a biological response (i.e. is without intrinsic activity). A drug acceptor as it has been formulated during the last few years is similarly a receptive site at a biological macromolecule involved in the biological function of a given class of drugs and might have a similar degree of specificity as well as the ability to bind agonists and antagonists. However, for a drug acceptor, an endogenous ligand (agonist) is not present. Thus, the major difference between a receptor and a drug acceptor is the lack of a physiological function of the latter. Both drug receptors and acceptors are different from the term 'silent receptor', which means a binding site without any physiological response, regardless of whether the ligand is endogenous or a drug. Silent receptors are some binding sites on plasma or tissue proteins (Müller & Wollert, 1979) and can have very high degrees of binding specificity (Müller *et al.*, 1986*a, c*).

The need to differentiate between classical receptors and drug acceptors has been brought about by the development of direct binding techniques over the last 10 years. A very good example is the opiate receptor, which for several years was only a drug acceptor in our present terminology. However, its discovery has finally led to the identification of several classes of endogenous morphine-like compounds (endorphins), representing physiological agonists of these binding sites (Akil *et al.*, 1984). Thus, even using classical standards, the opiate binding sites represent true receptors. A similar approach has been tried since the discovery of specific

Table 1.4 *General criteria for drug acceptors or receptors*

In terms of general criteria a drug acceptor differs from a receptor only by the lack of the presence of an endogenous ligand.

1 Displacement by agonists and antagonists
2 Structural specificity and stereospecificity
3 Correlation between binding affinity and pharmacological potency
4 High affinity, saturability, and reversibility of ligand binding
5 Specific regional distribution or tissue specificity
6 Agonists elicit a specific biological response
7 Presence of an endogenous agonist

Source: Adapted from Laduron, 1984.

benzodiazepine binding sites in the mammalian CNS. However, as we will learn later on, up to now all attempts have failed to identify clearly endogenous ligands comparable to the endorphins. Due to these negative findings, several authors have speculated that the presence of highly selective binding sites for drugs must not in any case imply the presence of an endogenous agonist, especially if the drug binding site represents only a modulatory or regulating subunit of another neuronal system, like the benzodiazepine receptor as the modulatory part of the GABAergic synapse (Möhler, 1981; Karobath, 1983 (see § 4.2 and 4.3). To name these drug binding sites, the term 'drug acceptor' was created.

One of the major arguments for the presence of drug acceptors (with the properties given in Table 1.4) as regulatory units of other neuronal systems was the belief that such drug acceptors are commonly found in the body. The most impressive examples for such putative drug acceptors are summarized in Table 1.5. All exhibit a certain degree of binding specificity and function as regulatory units of other neuronal systems. However, if we look much closer at the major characteristics of these binding sites, the general concept of drug acceptors is more discredited than supported. For example, the local anaesthetic binding site of the nicotinic cholinergic receptor does not fulfil the specificity criteria in respect to ligand binding (Table 1.4) (Conti-Tronconi & Raftery, 1982). The digitalis binding site of the Na^+-K^+-ATPase very likely represents a

Table 1.5 *Putative examples for the presence of drug acceptors as modulatory units of other neuronal systems*

Binding site	Specific ligand	Biological function: modulation of	Endogenous agonist	Drug acceptor or receptor
Digitalis	[^{3}H]ouabain	Na^+-K^+-ATPase	Yes	Receptor
Local anaesthetic	Specific high-affinity ligand not known	Nicotinic cholinergic receptor	No	Neither of the two
Imipramine	[^{3}H]imipramine	Neuronal 5-HT uptake	Possibly yes	Receptor
Peripheral benzodiazepine	[^{3}H]Ro 5–4864	Ca^{2+}-channel	Possibly yes	Receptor
Calcium antagonist	[^{3}H]nitrendipine	Ca^{2+}-channel	Possibly yes	Receptor

receptor, since several groups have described the presence of endogenous digitalis-like ligands in the mammalian body (Fishman, 1979; Halperin *et al.*, 1983; Lichtstein *et al.*, 1985). The imipramine binding site of the presynaptic serotoninergic neuron (Davis, 1984) also seems to be rather a receptor than an acceptor, since some evidence exists for the presence of endogenous agonists (Barbaccia *et al.*, 1983; Langer *et al.*, 1984; Rehavi *et al.*, 1984). The peripheral benzodiazepine binding site seems to exhibit the properties of a silent receptor rather than of a drug acceptor. However, very recently a biological response of agonist binding and the presence of a putative endogenous ligand have been reported (Beaumont *et al.*, 1983; Mestre *et al.*, 1984, 1985) (see also §2.6.1.). Thus, this site might also represent a receptor rather than a drug receptor. The last examples are the calcium antagonist binding sites (Braunwald, 1982; Murphy *et al.*, 1983) which come close to what we regard as a drug receptor. However, even for some of these sites, evidence for the presence of endogenous ligands has been presented (Hanbauer & Sanna, 1986). Accordingly, these sites again might be receptors rather than acceptors. The final question raising doubts on the concept of the presence of specific drug acceptors is why the body should possess such sites if there is no use for them. Evolution is usually very economical and structures not needed are usually eliminated by the evolutionary process. This is not the case, for example, with the benzodiazepine receptor, which appears first at the step from non-vertebrates to vertebrates (see § 2.3) and is maintained from this time up to the human brain without any change of its properties. This would seem very unlikely to be the case if these sites had no physiological function. Taken together, we have little conclusive evidence for the general presence of drug acceptors in the mammalian body. On the other hand, the presence of such sites cannot generally be ruled out.

In the case of the specific benzodiazepine recognition sites of the vertebrate CNS, evidence for and against a role as classical receptor will be discussed in the present book.

2

General aspects of the benzodiazepine receptor

As already mentioned in the previous chapter, for many years of extensive clinical use of the benzodiazepines, their molecular mechanism of action remained a mystery. The first general concept to explain benzodiazepine activity in certain areas of the brain was presented by several groups at the December 1974 meeting of the American College of Neuropsychopharmacology held in Puerto Rico (Costa *et al.*, 1975; Fuxe *et al.*, 1975; Haefely *et al.*, 1975). It assumed that benzodiazepines enhance the activity of the inhibitory neurotransmitter GABA at pre- and post-synaptic nerve terminals. Although the evidence for this concept came from pharmacological, electrophysiological and biochemical experiments, the final mechanism by which benzodiazepines could enhance GABAergic neurotransmission remained unclear for several years. Nearly all classical mechanisms known to influence the synaptic activity of a neurotransmitter were subsequently investigated, but none could account for the effects of benzodiazepines on GABAergic neurotransmission, e.g. agonistic activity at the GABA receptor, enhancement of GABA synthesis, reduction of the synaptic GABA degradation, interference with the neuronal or glial cell uptake of GABA, and direct effects at the GABA gated chloride channel. Thus, although the concept of benzodiazepines as indirect GABA-mimetic drugs became more and more widely accepted, the final mechanism of the indirect GABA-mimetic activity still remained unknown. On the other hand, the major conclusion which could be drawn from all these negative data was that benzodiazepines obviously did not interact with one of the already-known specific functions of the GABAergic neuron. This could indicate a non-specific effect of benzodiazepines on neuronal function like stabilization of the neuronal membrane. This conclusion, however, was very strongly contradictory to several earlier findings regarding benzodiazepine activity.

1 Benzodiazepine activity is highly dependent on the specific chemical structure of the benzodiazepine molecule and only very small changes in the molecule can change a highly potent compound into a completely inactive one (Sternbach, 1973), e.g. the change from 2′-chlorodiazepam (highly potent) by 4′-chlorine substitution to 4′-chlorodiazepam (practically inactive) (see also Fig. 2.7). Such a structural specificity speaks strongly against a non-specific mechanism of action.

2 For some benzodiazepine derivatives, pharmacological activity is highly stereospecific, with the (S)-enantiomer usually being much more potent than the respective (R)-enantiomers (Haefely *et al.*, 1985). Again, stereoselectivity favours specific much more than non-specific mechanisms.

3 Benzodiazepine activity can be very potent, with ED_{50} values in experimental animals well below 1 mg/kg or with therapeutic doses in man less than 1 mg. Again, such a high potency at the molecular level argues much more strongly in favour of the presence of a specific than of a non-specific mechanism of action.

The final solution which combined the high degree of structural specificity of benzodiazepine activity and the possible indirect GABA-mimetic activity was rather simple. Initiated by the findings of specific high-affinity binding sites for opiates in the CNS, it was assumed that benzodiazepine activity was mediated at the neuronal level by a specific 'benzodiazepine receptor' or, better, by a specific benzodiazepine binding site, similar to the opiate receptors present in various areas of the nervous system. The first evidence for the presence of such a benzodiazepine binding site was published by Squires & Braestrup in 1977 and confirmed only a few months later by Möhler & Okada (1977). The concept of the benzodiazepine receptor was born. Today, the presence of a specific receptor for benzodiazepines and a few related drugs in the CNS is a generally accepted fact. The basic biochemical and pharmacological characteristics of these binding sites have been reviewed in detail by Haefely *et al.* (1981, 1985), Braestrup & Nielsen (1983) and Squires (1984).

2.1 Binding technology and terminology

Since most of the early evidence for the presence of benzodiazepine-specific binding sites in the CNS of many vertebrate species came from direct binding experiments using tritiated benzodiazepines as radioligands, some of the general features of the binding technology will be reviewed in this chapter. However, the aim of this part is not to give an overview of the biochemical and biophysical aspects of receptor binding, but to introduce the reader not familiar with these methods to the basic aspects of receptor binding terminology, since this will be used throughout the book. The reader more interested in the technical aspects of receptor binding methods should refer to the book by Yamamura *et al.* (1978) entitled *Neurotransmitter receptor binding*.

The basic aspects of receptor binding technology are very simple. All experiments start (Fig. 2.1) by incubating a given tissue fraction (usually a homogenate) with a radioligand of high specific activity. Carbon-14 is not used; nearly all binding assays are performed with tritiated or iodinated (^{125}I or ^{131}I) radioligands. The need for ligands with high specific activity (usually greater than 1 Ci/mmol) will be explained later. After incubating the tissue with the radioligand for a given time (optimal conditions and equilibrium time have to be determined), the free radioligand, e.g. the radioligand still in the incubation medium, is separated from the radioligand bound to the tissue. This can be done by rapid filtration or by centrifugation (Fig. 2.1). After separation, the radioligand bound to the tissue can be determined easily; e.g. in the case of a tritiated radioligand, this is done by liquid scintillation spectrometry.

While this is very simple, it is not such a simple matter to establish that this binding represents the binding of the radioligand to its putative

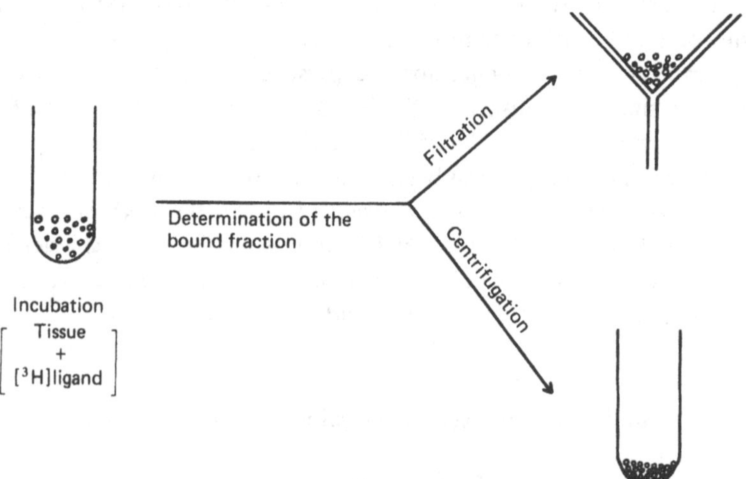

Fig. 2.1. Basic principles of receptor binding. The determination of the binding of a radioligand to a tissue homogenate by filtration or centrifugation (see text).

receptor. Unfortunately, practically all radioligands bind not only to their receptors, but also to different degrees to much less specific binding sites on the tissues investigated or even on the filters used for separating bound from free ligand. This unspecific or non-specific binding varies with the ligands and tissues used and can account for less than 5% up to more than 90% of total binding. It is quite conceivable that in the latter case total binding has nothing to do with receptor binding. Fortunately, though, receptor binding (also referred to as 'specific binding') and non-specific binding differ in some major aspects which make it possible to differentiate the two parts of total binding very easily. Specific (or receptor) binding of a given radioligand is usually of high affinity, which is the basis for the specific binding of the ligand to the receptor, but of low capacity, since the number of receptors is usually very low. By contrast, non-specific binding usually exhibits much lower affinities, but has a higher capacity, since the number of sites of most tissues able to bind ligands in a non-specific fashion is very much higher than that of specific receptors. Accordingly, if aliquot samples of the same tissue homogenate are incubated with the same concentration of the radioligand and with increasing concentrations of an unlabelled receptor ligand (Fig. 2.2), the cold ligand will preferentially displace the radioligand from the specific binding sites

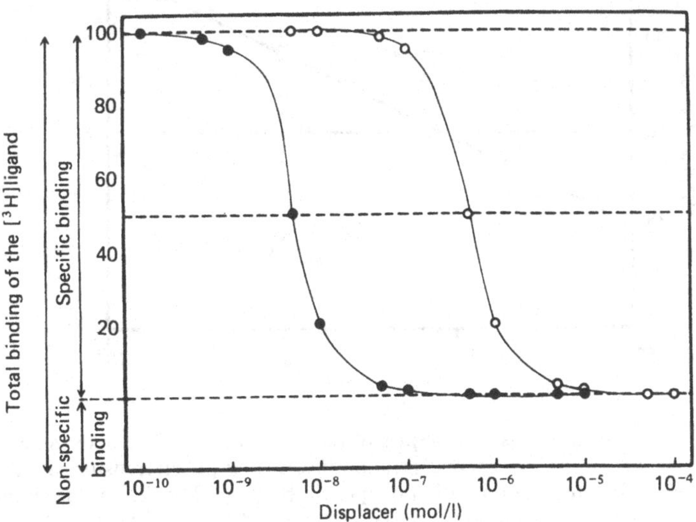

Fig. 2.2. Basic principles of receptor binding. The differentiation of total binding of a radioligand into specific (receptor-associated) and non-specific binding by displacement studies using unlabelled receptor ligands. For further details see text. (Adapted from Müller, 1981*a*.)

(receptor sites) up to a point at which all radioligand is displaced from the receptor sites. That part of total binding that is still found under such conditions will represent the non-specific binding, e.g. that part of total binding not associated with the respective receptor. Only if the concentration of the cold ligand is increased much further might displacement also take place from non-specific binding sites. This situation is not shown in the graph in Fig. 2.2. Another cold receptor ligand will show a similar displacement curve, reaching the same plateau value when all molecules of the radioligand are displaced from the receptor sites (Fig. 2.2). The cold ligands (displacers) differ in the concentrations needed for a similar displacement of the radioligand. This is indicated in Fig. 2.2 for the concentrations of two cold ligands needed to inhibit the specific binding of the radioligand by 50% (= inhibitory concentration 50%, IC_{50}). Such IC_{50} values are usually determined by plotting the data of S-shaped displacement curves in log-probit plots (Fig. 2.3), which usually result in straight lines. The exact value of the 50% point can be determined easily by regression analysis. For a given receptor binding system, such IC_{50} values are a direct measure of the affinities of the displacing, unlabelled

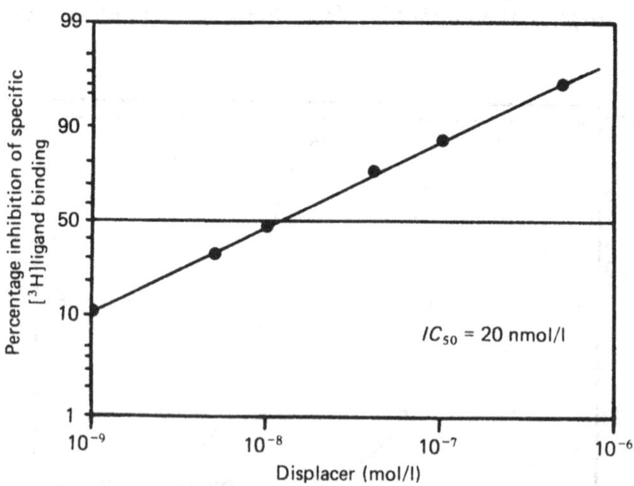

Fig. 2.3. Basic principles of receptor binding. The determination of an IC_{50} (inhibitory concentration 50%) by log-probit transformation of the data for the inhibition of specific binding. The IC_{50} value (inhibitory concentration 50%) can be transformed to the K_i value (inhibition constant) by use of the equation:

$$K_i = IC_{50}/(1 + c/K_D)$$

where c = the concentration of the radioligand used and K_D = its dissociation constant in the same system.

compounds for the receptor labelled by the radioligand used. If the inhibition of the radioligand binding is competitive, IC_{50} values can be transformed easily to inhibition constants, K_i, which represent a much better measure of receptor affinity, since the effect of the concentration of the radioligand is avoided (see the formula given in the legend to Fig. 2.3).

The scheme given in Fig. 2.2 illustrates another important aspect of receptor binding terminology, i.e. the use of a 'blank' to determine the amount of specific binding of the radioligand. As can be seen from the data given in the graph, at specific concentrations of both displacers, all radioligand molecules are displaced from the receptor sites, while non-specific binding is unaffected. This is the case at about 10^{-6}mol/l for the ligand indicated by the closed circles and at about 10^{-4}mol/l for the ligand indicated by the open circles. Thus, if, in parallel experiments, tissue samples are incubated with the radioligand only or with the same concentration of the radioligand as of a cold receptor ligand at such a 'blank' concentration, that amount of total binding associated with specific receptor binding can be determined easily from the difference between the two values for a large variety of different experimental conditions.

The most important example for the use of a blank is the determination of the maximal number of specific binding sites in a given tissue homogenate by saturation experiments (Fig. 2.4). For such experiments, aliquots of the same tissue homogenate are incubated in parallel experiments with increasing concentrations of the radioligand either alone or in the presence of a high concentration of a cold receptor ligand (blank), resulting in data for total and non-specific binding respectively. The difference between the two values gives for each of the concentrations of the radioligand the amount of specific binding. As can be seen from the data given in Fig. 2.4*a*, specific binding of the radioligand becomes saturated at relatively low concentrations, while non-specific binding increases linearly with the concentration of the radioligand used. To saturate non-specific binding, much higher concentrations of the radioligand would be needed.

Figure 2.4*a* further illustrates that the ratio between specific and non-specific binding becomes smaller with increasing concentrations of the radioligand. Accordingly, in order to obtain a satisfactory signal to noise ratio, binding studies have to be done at very low concentrations of the radioligand, where more is bound to the receptor than to non-specific binding sites. This need to work at very low concentrations of the radioligand explains why ligands with high specific activity are needed for such receptor binding experiments (see above).

Binding data for specific binding as obtained by such saturation experiments are usually transformed according to the mass law action into a Scatchard plot (Scatchard, 1949), where the maximal number of binding sites for the system investigated can be determined from the extrapolation of the curve to the abscissa (Fig. 2.4*b*). If the data result in a straight line as indicated in this graph, evidence is present for an interaction of the radioligand with a single homogeneous population of binding sites. If the

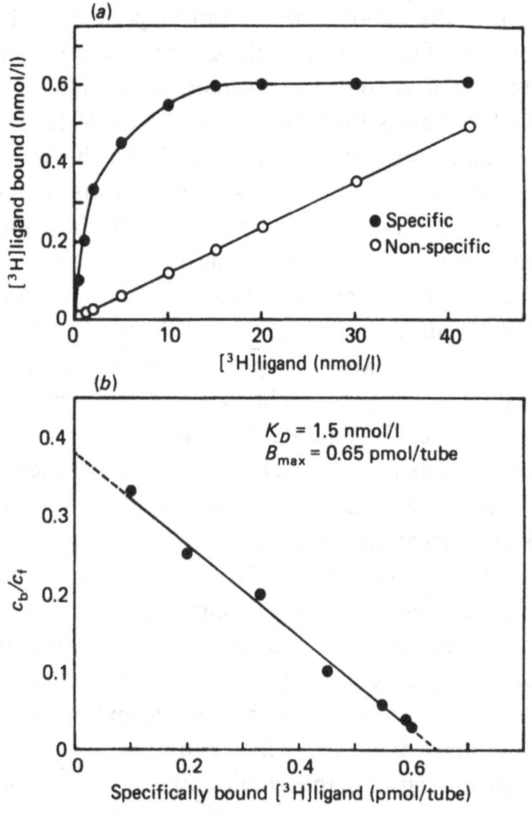

Fig. 2.4. Basic principles of receptor binding.
(*a*) The dependence of specific and non-specific binding on total ligand concentration.
(*b*) Scatchard transformation of the data for specific binding according to the equation:

$$B/F = \frac{B_{max} - B}{K_D}$$

Where B = the concentration of bound ligand, F = the concentration of free ligand, B_{max} = the maximum number of binding sites, and K_D = the dissociation constant. c_b and c_f are the concentrations of bound and free ligand respectively. For further details see text. (Adapted from Müller, 1981*a*.)

data result in a curved line, the radioligand might interact with at least two populations of sites exhibiting different affinities for the radioligand. In the case of a single population of binding sites, the dissociation constant (K_D) of the radioligand–receptor complex can be determined from the slope of the straight line (Fig. 2.4*b*). For practical considerations, the dissociation constant gives that concentration of the radioligand which is needed to occupy 50% of the receptors in a given system. If the same compound is used for the determination of a K_D value as well as a K_i value, the values should be similar. Both are measures of receptor affinity. The lower the K_D or K_i values, the higher the affinity of the ligand for the receptor.

In the case of the benzodiazepine receptor, such simple techniques have been used to identify the population of specific binding sites in the CNS of many species including man. In most cases, tritiated diazepam or tritiated flunitrazepam have been used as radioligands. Some other tritiated benzodiazepines (clonazepam, meclonazepam) and tritiated benzodiazepine receptor ligands (Ro 15–1788, some β-carbolines) have also been used.

2.2 Saturability and regional distribution

2.2.1 *Saturability*

Using the basic techniques described above, saturable specific but not saturable non-specific binding of tritiated benzodiazepine derivatives (mostly [^{3}H]diazepam and [^{3}H]flunitrazepam) has been found in homogenates of CNS tissue of a large variety of species investigated, similar to the example of the binding of [^{3}H]flunitrazepam to a crude homogenate of bovine retina (Fig. 2.5). As in this example, the maximum number of binding sites (B_{max} or receptor density) is usually within the range of less than 1 up to a few picomoles per milligramme membrane protein, a concentration range found for several other receptors for neurotransmitters or drugs in the CNS. Some early findings about benzodiazepine receptor densities in various tissues are summarized in Table 2.1. From such data, it has been estimated that whole rat brain contains about 10^{13} benzodiazepine receptors per gramme wet weight (Müller, 1981*a*).

Even when assayed in the same brain region of the same species, considerable differences have been found for B_{max} values by different authors, due to small differences in binding technology. The major reason for these differences is the different degrees of purification of the membrane fractions used for the binding assay. It is conceivable that density, given in pmol/mg protein, will differ according to whether a highly purified membrane fraction enriched in receptors or a crude whole brain homogenate, where all soluble cytosol proteins are still present, is used for the assay. Therefore, B_{max} values can be used to investigate differences of benzodiazepine receptor density only if all assay conditions, including the tissue preparation, are identical. If they are identical, the determination of B_{max} values by Scatchard analysis represents a valuable tool to

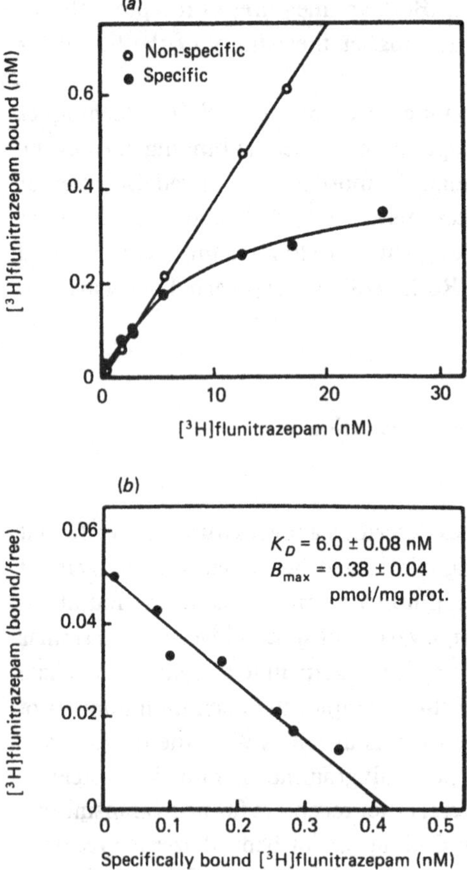

Fig. 2.5. Saturation of specific [^{3}H]flunitrazepam binding to bovine retina homogenates.
(*a*) The relationship between specific and non-specific binding and total ligand concentration. This example shows clearly the increasing ratio between the two parts of total binding with increasing ligand concentration.
(*b*) Scatchard analysis of specific binding. Data for B_{max} and K_D are the means of four identical experiments. (Data are taken from Borbe *et al.*, 1980.)

demonstrate even small differences of benzodiazepine receptor densities in related tissues.

Using this method, the differences in benzodiazepine receptor densities between the cerebella of normal and *Lurcher* mutant mice have been determined (Fig. 2.6). The data indicate that the density of the benzodiazepine receptors in the *Lurcher* mutant is about 55% lower than that found in the control mice. Since this neurological mutant is characterized by a loss of more than 99.5% of the Purkinje and about 90% of the granule cells, the data suggest that the density of benzodiazepine receptors on cerebellar neurons other than Purkinje and granule cells is less than the density on these two types of cerebellar cell. However, if the data presented in Fig. 2.6 are calculated in terms of maximal number of benzodiazepine receptors per cerebellum, the number of receptors on the *Lurcher* cerebellum is reduced by about 90% relative to the controls (Table 2.2). Thus, about 90% of the benzodiazepine receptors of the mouse cerebellum are localized on the Purkinje and granule cells. These findings

Table 2.1 *Determination of benzodiazepine receptor density* I

Some early findings about the density of the benzodiazepine receptor in CNS tissues of several species.

Tissue	Ligand	K_D (nmol/l)	B_{max} (pmol/mg protein)	Reference
Rat cortex	[^{3}H]diaz	3.5	0.81	Möhler & Okada (1977)
Whole rat brain	[^{3}H]diaz	6.1	0.95	Müller *et al.* (1978*a*)
Rat spinal cord	[^{3}H]diaz	8.1	0.48	Müller *et al.* (1978*b*)
Bovine retina	[^{3}H]FNT	6.0	0.38	Borbe *et al.* (1980)
Rat forebrain	[^{3}H]diaz	14.8	0.36	Bossmann *et al.* (1978)
Human cortex	[^{3}H]diaz	3.5	0.86	Braestrup *et al.* (1977)
Human cortex	[^{3}H]diaz	6.0	1.20	Möhler & Okada (1978)
Human spinal cord	[^{3}H]diaz	7.0	0.21	Braestrup *et al.* (1977)
Human cortex	[^{3}H]FNT	2.8	0.89	Speth *et al.* (1978*a*)

indicate the critical nature of the reference used for the determination of changes in receptor densities: data have to be evaluated very carefully if apparent changes in receptor density are not to reflect changes in the reference used.

Beside these methodological problems, overwhelming evidence has been presented that benzodiazepine receptors can be saturated with relatively

Table 2.2 *Determination of benzodiazepine receptor density* II

Saturation of specific [^{3}H]flunitrazepam binding in cerebellar homogenates from normal and *Lurcher* mutant mice. B_{max} values, as taken from Scatchard plots (see Fig. 2.4), were calculated either in relation to mg membrane protein or as binding per cerebellum. The size of the *Lurcher* cerebellum is only about 30% of that of the controls due to the loss of Purkinje and granule cells. The data in parentheses indicate the B_{max} of the *Lurcher* mice as a percentage of the B_{max} of the controls.

	K_D (nmol/l)	B_{max} (pmol/mg protein)	B_{max} (pmol/cerebellum)
Controls	10.2	1.14	4.98
Lurcher	15.3	0.51 (44)	0.56 (11)

Source: Data are taken from Sauer *et al.* (1984).

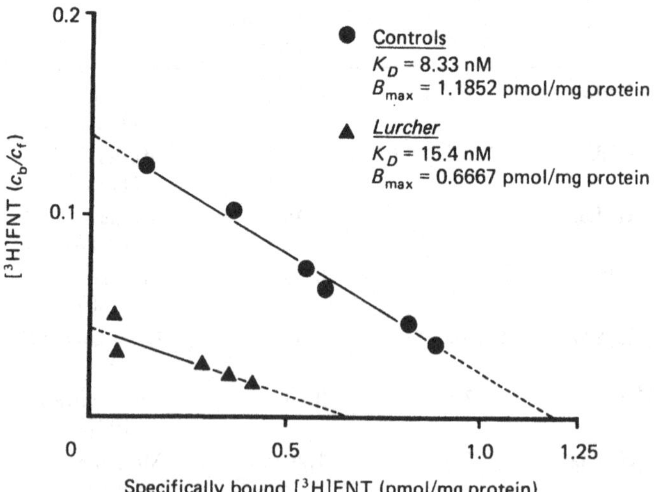

Fig. 2.6. Saturation of specific [^{3}H]flunitrazepam binding in homogenates of the cerebellum of normal and *Lurcher* mutant mice. c_b and c_f are the concentrations of bound and free ligands respectively. Data are presented as a Scatchard analysis. (Adapted from Sauer *et al.*, 1984.)

small concentrations of the radioligands used, indicating the presence of a defined concentration or density of these receptors in each tissue investigated.

2.2.2 *Regional distribution*

Using the general binding methods described above, the distribution of benzodiazepine receptors has been investigated in many species. As a general rule, benzodiazepine receptors are widely but unevenly distributed over all parts of the CNS, including the retina, pineal gland and pituitary, but cannot be found outside the CNS. As an example, the distribution of benzodiazepine receptors within the rat brain is given in Table 2.3, indicating high densities in cortical areas and in areas of the limbic system, and intermediate densities in most other areas, except the brain stem and spinal cord where low densities are present. Similar but not identical distributions have been found in all other species investigated so far including man (see Chapter 5). During the last few years, great progress has been made in studies of the distribution of benzodiazepine receptors at the intraregional level using light-microscopic autoradiographic methods (for review see Haefely *et al.*, 1985). These studies have shown that benzodiazepine receptors are not evenly distributed over a given high or low density area, but are localized on specific structures of a given brain area only, e.g. within the low-density spinal cord benzodiazepine receptors are mainly present in the dorsal horn and in Lamina X around the central canal (Haefely *et al.*, 1985). Up to now, no differences have been found in the general characteristics of benzodiazepine receptors in all the brain areas and species investigated, except that the relative fraction of putative BZ_1 and BZ_2 receptor subclasses might differ between brain areas and species (see § 2.5).

As already mentioned, benzodiazepine receptors have been found only in the CNS of all the species investigated so far. In order to indicate this fact and to distinguish these sites from the peripheral benzodiazepine binding sites (see § 2.6.1), benzodiazepine receptors are also termed 'brain-specific benzodiazepine binding sites'. Perhaps the only exception to this known so far is the possible presence of benzodiazepine receptors in bovine adrenal chromaffin cells (Kataoka *et al.*, 1984). Similar to the situation of those in the CNS, the benzodiazepine receptors of the bovine adrenal chromaffin cells are part of a functioning GABA receptor–benzodiazepine receptor–chloride channel complex, as indicated by recent findings using the patch–clamp technique (Bormann & Clapham, 1985). Whether these sites are also present on adrenal chromaffin cells of other species and

Table 2.3 *Regional distribution of the benzodiazepine receptor in rat brain*

The data represent the relative densities (calculated with reference to mg membrane protein) using the value for the brain region with the highest density (olfactory bulb) as 100%.

Region	Relative density (%)
Cerebral cortex	
Frontal	98
Occipital	60
Rhinencephalon	
Olfactory bulb	100
Olfactory tubercle	14
Hippocampus, dorsal	80
Hippocampus, ventral	67
Amygdala, anterior	78
Amygdala, posterior	71
Cingulate cortex	73
Septum	37
Nucleus accumbens	42
Basal ganglia	
Caudata/putamen	35
Globus pallidus	32
Diencephalon	
Medial forebrain bundle, anterior	60
Medial forebrain bundle, posterior	34
Preoptic area	50
Mammillary body	45
Arcuate nucleus	38
Ventromedial nucleus	36
Anterior ventral nucleus (thalamus)	31
Ventral nucleus (thalamus)	14
Medial nucleus (thalamus)	22
Medial geniculate	32
Lateral geniculate	18
Median eminence	22
Ventral tegmental area	17
Mesencephalon	
Substantia nigra	18
Interpeduncular nucleus	21
Red nucleus	56
Inferior colliculus	60
Superior colliculus	59
Reticular formation	53
Central gray	53

Table 2.3 (*cont.*)

Region	Relative density (%)
Metencephalon	
Cerebellar cortex	29
Cerebellar nuclei	12
Pons	13
Locus coeruleus	24
Mylencephalon	
Medulla	18
Spinal cord	
Cervical cord	10
Pituitary	1

Source: Data are adapted from Speth *et al.* (1980).

whether they have any functional relevance for the pharmacological properties of the benzodiazepines remain to be investigated.

2.2.3 *Cellular and subcellular distribution*

A variety of experimental evidence suggests that benzodiazepine receptors are usually located on neuronal cell membranes of the CNS. Their presence on glial cells is still controversial. Some of the early findings in this respect possibly indicate the presence of peripheral benzodiazepine binding sites rather than brain-specific benzodiazepine receptors on glial cells (see § 2.6.1). Within the neuron, the majority of the benzodiazepine receptors are localized at the soma membranes, but some might also be present at the membranes of dendrites and synaptic terminals. Evidence for an intracellular localization of benzodiazepine receptors is only marginal, possibly indicating synthesis of the receptor protein in the cell.

Since benzodiazepine receptor function is associated with the GABA receptor, it seems important to know to what extent benzodiazepine receptor distribution parallels that of the GABA receptor. Several lines of evidence suggest that many GABA receptors in the CNS are not associated with benzodiazepine receptors. On the other hand, most if not all benzodiazepine receptors seem to be associated with GABA receptors, which agrees very well with the concept of benzodiazepines being indirectly GABA-mimetic drugs. More details of the cellular and subcellular distribution of the benzodiazepine receptor are given in the reviews of Haefely *et al.* (1981, 1985), Braestrup & Nielsen (1983), and Squires (1984).

2.3 Phylogenetic and ontogenetic development

The phylogenetic development of the benzodiazepine receptor has been investigated in detail by Fernholm *et al.* (1979) and Nielsen *et al.* (1978). Benzodiazepine receptors appear relatively late in evolution, approximately at the step from invertebrates to vertebrates. However, these receptors are not yet present in the brains of some lower fishes like lamprey and shark, but are present in the brains of higher fishes like eel and codfish. Beginning from this point of evolution, these receptors have been found in the brains of Amphibia (e.g. toad, frog), of Reptilia (e.g. turtle, lizard), of Aves (e.g. pigeon, hen), and of all Mammalia investigated so far. Apart from some findings in fishes, the major properties of the benzodiazepine receptor are the same in all these species investigated, indicating that possible changes by mutation have been repaired during evolution from fishes up to man. Very interestingly, the phylogenetic development of the benzodiazepine receptor is quite different from that of the GABA receptor. GABA receptors appear much earlier in evolution and are already present in the brains of lower vertebrates like the Cyclostomata and Chondrichthyes (which include lamprey and shark) and in the brains of some invertebrates such as some Crustacea (e.g. lobster), all of which are devoid of benzodiazepine receptors (Nielsen *et al.*, 1978; Fernholm *et al.*, 1979).

The ontogenetic development of the benzodiazepine receptor has been studied in the rat and the mouse brain using tissue binding and autoradiographic techniques (see Braestrup & Nielsen, 1983, and Haefely *et al.*, 1985). Benzodiazepine receptors are first detected after 14 to 16 days' gestation, reach about 30% of the adult level at birth, and reach the adult level about 3 weeks after birth. The receptors appear first in the phylogenetically older areas, like the spinal cord and lower brain stem, and spread into the other brain areas in a sequence possibly linked with cell differentiation.

Some studies indicate that the development of the benzodiazepine receptor parallels that of the GABA receptor, while other reports indicate a faster development of the benzodiazepine receptor than of the GABA receptor. Since not all GABA receptors are linked to benzodiazepine receptors, even the latter findings do not necessarily suggest that the ontogenetic development of the different parts of the benzodiazepine receptor–GABA receptor–chloride channel complex is different.

2.4 Substrate specificity

Biologically active receptors are built to recognize and bind only one physiological ligand (neurotransmitter or hormone) out of the large variety of compounds present in our bodies. Thus, receptors usually have a very pronounced structural specificity. This is also the case for the benzodiazepine receptor, which binds only certain biologically active benzodiazepine derivatives with high affinity (although a few exceptions will be referred to later on). The high degree of structural specificity of several diazepam derivatives is demonstrated in Fig. 2.7. While the step from diazepam to desmethyldiazepam has little effect on the receptor affinity and the biological activity, the introduction of a chlorine atom in position 2′ of the β-benzene ring profoundly changes both affinity and biological activity (chlordesmethyldiazepam in Fig. 2.7). Very interestingly, if the chlorine atom is introduced into position 4′ of the β-benzene ring instead, receptor affinity is reduced by many orders of magnitude and biological activity is practically lost (Ro 5–4864 in Fig. 2.7). Similar structure–binding and structure–activity relationships have been deduced for many benzodiazepine derivatives (for a review, see Haefely *et al.*, 1985). The general conclusion that can be drawn is that only biologically active

Substance	R_1	R_2	R_3	IC_{50} (nmol/l) [^{3}H]Ro 5–4864	[^{3}H]FNT	*R*	Potency
Diazepam	$-CH_3$	phenyl	–H	29	17	1.7	+ + +
Desmethyldiazepam	–H	phenyl	–H	9000	25	360.0	+ + +
Temazepam	$-CH_3$	phenyl	–OH	550	37	15.0	+ + +
Tetrazepam	$-CH_3$	cyclohexenyl	–H	38	75	0.5	+ +
Ro 5–4864	$-CH_3$	4′-Cl-phenyl	–H	4	73000	0.00005	0
Chlordesmethyldiazepam	–H	2′-Cl-phenyl	–H	2500	0.3	8300.0	+ + + +

Fig. 2.7. The relationship between the affinity of several diazepam derivatives for the benzodiazepine receptor as indicated by the IC_{50} against specific [^{3}H]flunitrazepam ([^{3}H]FNT) binding or the affinity for the peripheral benzodiazepine binding site as indicated by the IC_{50} against specific [^{3}H]Ro 5–4864 binding and their pharmacological potency (protection against pentetrazole-induced convulsions) (+ + + + very potent, 0 without effect). *R* represents the ratio IC_{50} [^{3}H]Ro 5–4864: IC_{50} [^{3}H]FNT. The pharmacological data are taken from Haefely *et al.* (1985) and the binding data from our laboratory.

Table 2.4 *A comparison between benzodiazepine receptor affinity and elimination half-life in man*

The drugs represent the 24 benzodiazepine derivatives currently on the market in West Germany (*Rote Liste*, 1986). Oxazolam is a prodrug; only desmethyldiazepam is present as an active component in human plasma after oral administration (Klotz, 1984).

Benzodiazepine	IC_{50} (nmol/l)	$t_{1/2}$ (h)
Alprazolam	20	10–18
Bromazepam	18	12–24
Brotiazolam	1	4– 8
Camazepam	900	10–24
Chlordiazepoxid	350	10–18*
Clobazam	130	10–30*
Clonazepam	2	24–56
Clorazepate	59	2– 3*
Clotiazepam	2[a]	3–15
Diazepam	8	30–45*
Flunitrazepam	4	10–25
Flurazepam	15	2*
Ketazolam	1 300[b]	1.5*
Lorazepam	4	10–18
Lormetazepam	4[c]	9–15
Medazepam	870	2*
Midazolam	5	1– 3
Nitrazepam	10	20–50
Oxazepam	18	5–18
Oxazolam	10 000[c]	—
Desmethyldiazepam	9	50–80
Prazepam	110	1– 3*
Temazepam	16	6–16
Tetrazepam	34	12
Triazolam	4	2– 4

Notes:
*The elimination half-life of the active drug is much longer due to the presence of active, slowly eliminated metabolites.

Source: Data for the inhibitory concentrations 50% against specific [^{3}H]diazepam binding (IC_{50}) are taken from Haefely *et al.* (1985) except for the following:

benzodiazepine derivatives bind to the benzodiazepine receptor. This is also true for several examples of stereospecific binding (Haefely *et al.*, 1985).

However, the observation that only the active benzodiazepines bind to the benzodiazepine receptor does not suggest that all active benzodiazepines bind to the receptor with similar affinity. This is shown by the receptor affinities of the 24 benzodiazepine derivatives presently on the market in West Germany, whose IC_{50} values vary by more than three orders of magnitude (Table 2.4). But again, the receptor is very selective and receptor affinity correlates closely with biological activity, as we will see in the next chapter. The very high substrate specificity of the benzodiazepine receptor has been further substantiated by the findings that, out of a large variety of different drugs, neurotransmitters and other biomolecules, only pharmacologically active benzodiazepines bind to this receptor system (Braestrup & Squires, 1978; Mackerer *et al.*, 1978). Again, binding specificity was strongly correlated with biological activity. However, the general rule that only pharmacologically active benzodiazepines bind to the benzodiazepine receptor is not without exception. Some putative endogenous ligands also bind to this receptor with considerable affinity (see Table 6.4) and, as we will hear in § 3.4, high-affinity benzodiazepine receptor ligands have also been synthesised as pure antagonists of the benzodiazepine receptor. Moreover, a few non-benzodiazepine drugs with benzodiazepine-related pharmacological properties have been synthesised, which bind to the benzodiazepine receptor and whose pharmacological properties are mediated by this mechanism (Fig. 2.8). However, most of these compounds are not full benzodiazepine receptor agonists but rather partial agonists or mixed agonists–antagonists (see § 4.4). Despite the rather complicated pharmacology of all benzodiazepine receptor ligands presently available, in all cases there is a very good relationship between binding and biological activity. In other words, the receptor recognizes only those substances which have relevant effects on receptor function, which is a major characteristic of any physiologically relevant receptor system.

Source Notes to Table 2.4 (*cont.*)
[a]Data from Möhler & Okada (1977)
[b]Data from Blaschke *et al.* (1986)
[c]Data from Braestrup & Nielsen (1983).
Data for the elimination half-lives ($t_{1/2}$) are taken from the review by Klotz (1984).

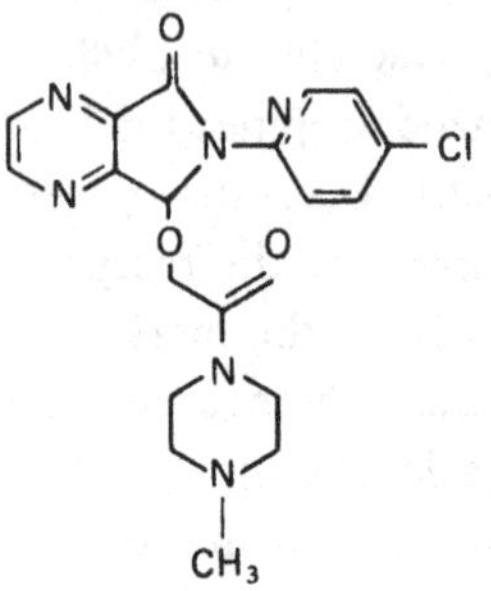

Zopiclone
(IC_{50} = 31)

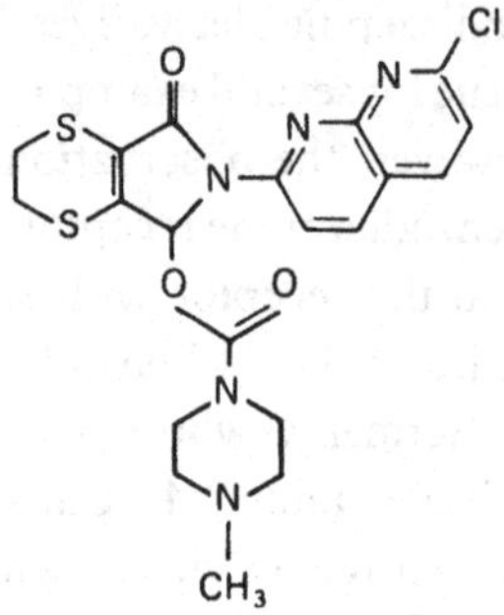

Suriclone
(IC_{50} = 2.1)

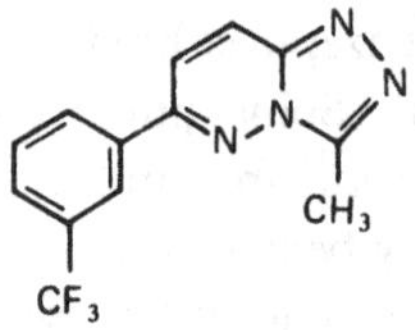

CI 218 872
(IC_{50} = 120)

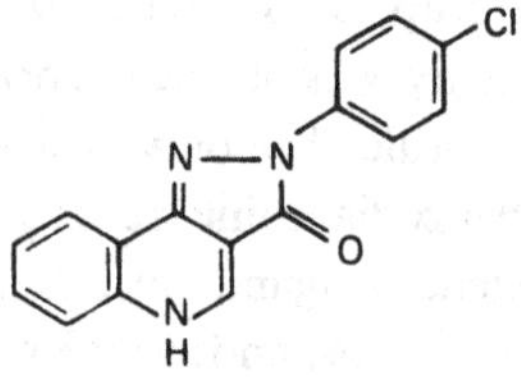

CGS 9896
(IC_{50} = 0.7)

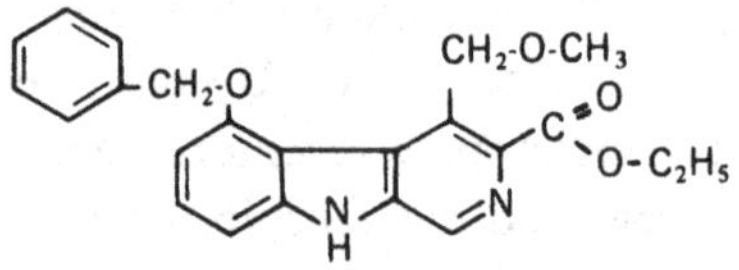

ZK 91296
(IC_{50} = 1)

Fig. 2.8. Structural formulae and benzodiazepine receptor affinity (given as IC_{50} value against specific [^{3}H]flunitrazepam in nmol/l) of several non-benzodiazepine drugs acting through the benzodiazepine receptor (benzodiazepine-like agonists). Out of these compounds, only zopiclone has been introduced into clinical practice and is available as a hypnotic in France.

2.5 Receptor subclasses

Until recently, all binding experiments made with the classical benzodiazepine derivatives (for examples, see Table 2.4) indicated the presence of only one class or population of benzodiazepine receptors with similar properties for all brain areas in all species investigated so far. Thus, using classical benzodiazepine derivatives, it is not possible to differentiate the homogeneous population of benzodiazepine receptors into receptor subclasses. However, evidence has been presented during recent years that a few non-benzodiazepine ligands of the benzodiazepine receptor are able to discriminate between two subclasses of the receptor, one of which binds these ligands with considerably higher affinity than the other. These two putative benzodiazepine receptor subclasses have tentatively been termed BZ_1 and BZ_2 receptors. Benzodiazepine receptor ligands binding with some degree of specificity to the BZ_1 subclass include the triazolopyridazine Cl 218 872 (see Fig. 2.8) and some β-carboline derivatives like propyl β-carboline-3-carboxylate (PrCC). Using one of these compounds as tritiated receptor ligands, the density of the BZ_1 subclass can be determined in a given tissue by saturation experiments (see Fig. 2.9 and Table 2.5). Since a specific ligand of the BZ_2 receptor subclass is not yet known, their concentration can presently be determined only indirectly by the difference between the density found for the BZ_1 subclass and the density of the total receptor population as determined by binding studies using a non-selective ligand, e.g. [^{3}H]FNT (Fig. 2.9 and Table 2.5).

Using similar homogenate experiments or related autoradiographic techniques, many aspects of both benzodiazepine receptor subclasses have been determined (Braestrup & Nielsen, 1983; Haefely *et al.*, 1985). Both subclasses show variations in their relative distribution between brain areas and usually have a distinct regional distribution in the brain (see the data for bovine brain in Table 2.5, and the more detailed data for rat brain in Table 2.6). While the tendency for relatively high densities of the BZ_1 subclass in the cerebellum and considerably lower relative densities in most other brain areas has been confirmed for many other species, divergent findings have also been reported (Sauer *et al.*, 1984). The subclasses might also differ in respect to their ontogenetic development (Haefely *et al.*, 1985; Sieghart, 1985).

The concept of the presence of at least two benzodiazepine receptor subclasses is also supported by biochemical data indicating the presence of different receptor proteins, one of which, with an apparent molecular weight of 51 000 (P_{51} protein), is possibly associated specifically with the BZ_1 subclass (for a review, see Sieghart, 1985). One the other hand, the

Table 2.5 *Distribution of putative benzodiazepine receptor subclasses in the bovine CNS*

The data indicate the total number of benzodiazepine receptors as determined by the B_{max} values for specific [^{3}H]FNT binding and the number of putative BZ_1 receptors as determined by the B_{max} values for specific [^{3}H]PrCC binding. The numbers in parentheses indicate BZ_1 receptors as a percentage of the total population (taken from Fehske *et al.*, 1982).

Bovine brain region	B_{max} (fmol/mg protein)	
	[^{3}H]FNT	[^{3}H]PrCC
Cerebellum	712	565 (79%)
Cortex	1650	1018 (62%)
Hippocampus	1322	787 (60%)
Retina	692	437 (63%)

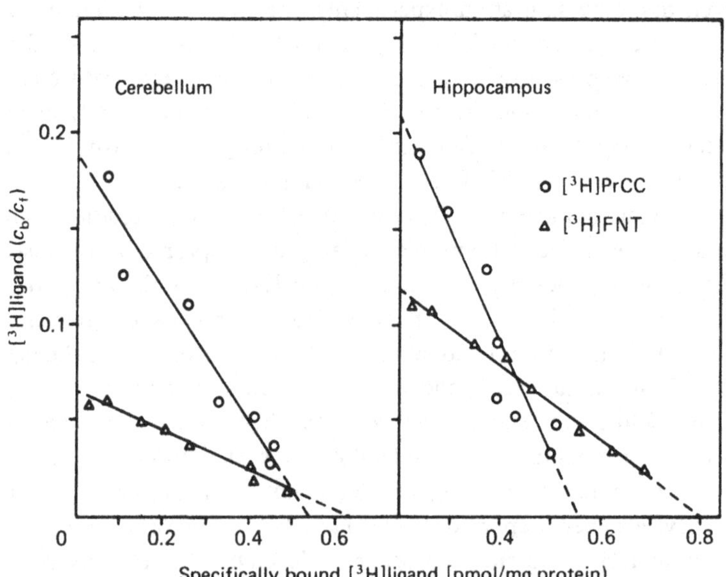

Fig. 2.9. Scatchard analysis of specific [^{3}H]FNT and specific [^{3}H]PrCC binding in two areas of the bovine brain, indicating that specific [^{3}H]PrCC binding labels fewer sites in both areas. The PrCC sensitive sites are usually designated as BZ_1 receptors, while the sites not sensitive to PrCC but labelled by [^{3}H]FNT are designated as BZ_2 sites. (Data are taken from Fehske *et al.* 1982.)

concept of the presence of at least two subclasses of the benzodiazepine receptor has been questioned by findings that the preferential affinity of some ligands for the BZ_1 subclass is mainly present at 4 °C (the temperature at which most binding experiments are carried out for practical reasons) and that these differences nearly disappear when the binding experiments are carried out at 37 °C (for reviews, see Ehlert *et al.*, 1983; Martin *et al.*, 1983; Sieghart, 1985). It has been suggested that the differences found by binding experiments might indicate the presence of different conformational states of the same receptor rather than the presence of two different receptor subclasses. This model, however, cannot also explain all of the different findings described above. Thus, Sieghart (1985) proposed the presence of two biochemically different benzodiazepine receptor subclasses, each capable of assuming two different conformational states.

Although we have rather sophisticated data about two biochemically distinct benzodiazepine receptor subclasses, the physiological or pharmacological significance of these putative subclasses is not known. The hypothesis that BZ_1-selective compounds like Cl 218 872 possess a

Table 2.6 *Distribution of putative benzodiazepine receptor subclasses in the rat CNS*

The data indicate the relative proportion of BZ_1 receptors out of the total benzodiazepine receptor population as labelled by the specific binding of [^{3}H]FNT.

Brain region	BZ_1 receptors as a percentage of the total receptor population
Cerebellum	100 (definition)
Medial cortex	84
Pons	81
Occipital cortex	81
Thalamus	80
Frontal cortex	78
Bulbus olfactorius	78
Corpus striatum	62
Hippocampus	59
Nucleus accumbens	57
Hypothalamus	57
Whole forebrain	69

Source: Data are taken from Braestrup & Nielsen (1983).

pharmacological spectrum different from that of the classical benzodiazepines (anxiolytic and anticonvulsive but with fewer sedative and muscle-relaxant properties), as originally pointed out by Lippa *et al.* (1979), could not be substantiated in subsequent investigations (Oakley *et al.*, 1984). Thus, even if these subclasses of the benzodiazepine receptor do exist, it remains to be demonstrated whether they mediate different pharmacological effects of benzodiazepine receptor ligands (Hirsch *et al.*, 1985). Accordingly, attempts to promote some newer benzodiazepine derivatives, like quazepam, as drugs with high pharmacological selectivity due to their in vitro preference for the BZ_1 subclass (Ongini & Barnett, 1984) must at present be viewed very critically.

2.6 Other high-affinity benzodiazepine binding sites

As discussed above, saturability, high-affinity and pronounced substrate specificity are important characteristics of the benzodiazepine receptor. However, for the final identification of these binding sites as the primary locus of benzodiazepine activity, many additional parameters (see Chapter 3) are important. Thus, binding specificity is one but not a sufficient criterion on which to characterize a specific receptor. As examples of high-affinity binding sites not representing functionally relevant drug acceptors or even drug receptors, the properties of the peripheral benzodiazepine binding site, of the micromolar benzodiazepine binding site, and of the indole and benzodiazepine binding site of human serum albumin will be reviewed briefly.

2.6.1 *The peripheral benzodiazepine binding site*

Even in their first publication about the presence of specific benzodiazepine binding sites in rat brain, Braestrup & Squires (1977) also demonstrated the presence of specific and high-affinity benzodiazepine binding sites in several peripheral organs. However, these sites exhibited different substrate specificity, since the highly potent benzodiazepine derivative clonazepam showed only a very weak affinity for these sites. Similar sites have subsequently been identified in most peripheral tissues investigated, including platelets and white blood cells. All these early studies used tritiated diazepam or tritiated flunitrazepam as radioligands. However, after the introduction of tritiated 4′-chlorodiazepam ([^{3}H]Ro 5–4864), a specific ligand for these sites became available with negligible affinity for the brain-specific benzodiazepine receptor (see Fig. 2.7). By the use of this radioligand, it was possible to identify so-called 'peripheral benzodiazepine binding sites' not only in peripheral organs but also in CNS tissues of many species (for reviews, see Squires, 1984, and Haefely *et al.*, 1985). These sites differ from the benzodiazepine receptor with respect to their regional distribution, with highest densities found in the olfactory bulb, the pineal, the neurohypophysis, ependyma and choroid plexus, with respect to their cellular distribution, with a possibly specific association of these sites with glial cells, and with respect to their phylogenetic development, since these sites are probably specific for mammalian vertebrates (Bolger *et al.*, 1985). The most important difference between the central benzodiazepine receptors and the peripheral benzodiazepine binding sites is their completely different substrate specificity (Wang *et al.*, 1984) which, however, is typical for these sites and does not differ between the different organs and between the different species investigated. Very importantly, there is no correlation between affinity for these sites and benzodiazepine activity in man and other animals, as can be seen from the examples of diazepam derivatives in Fig. 2.7 and has been demonstrated for many more benzodiazepine derivatives (Squires, 1984; Haefely *et al.*, 1985).

While there is presently little doubt that the peripheral benzodiazepine binding sites are not involved in any of the relevant pharmacological or clinical properties of the benzodiazepines, some controversy exists as to whether there is any pharmacological effect mediated by these sites. It has been suggested that some central effects of Ro 5–4864 (anxiogenic and proconvulsive), acting as a specific agonist, are mediated by these sites and can be antagonized by the isoquinoline derivative PK 11195, acting as a specific antagonist (Bénavidès *et al.*, 1984*a*; Mizoule *et al.*, 1985). These findings, however, are not undisputed and it has been suggested alternatively that the central effects of both drugs are mediated by sites different from the peripheral benzodiazepine binding sites in the CNS (Pellow & File, 1984; File & Pellow, 1985).

Outside the CNS, it has been suggested that the peripheral benzodiazepine binding sites are associated with calcium channels in the guinea-pig heart (Mestre *et al.*, 1984, 1985). This conclusion, however, has also been questioned very recently (Holck & Osterrieder, 1985) due to contradictory electrophysiological observations.

PK 11195 was found to inhibit in very low concentration the stimulatory activity of several benzodiazepines on the chemotaxis of human monocytes, an effect possibly mediated by peripheral benzodiazepine binding sites present on these cells (Ruff *et al.*, 1985). It has been speculated by the authors that this effect might represent one of the possible mechanisms connecting the CNS with the immune system.

In conclusion, while little doubt exists that these sites represent very specific recognition sites for several benzodiazepines and related compounds, it is not yet known whether they should be classified as pharmacologically inactive 'silent receptors', as pharmacologically active drug acceptors, or even as physiological receptors of some not yet further characterized endogenous ligands which have yet to be fully characterized (Beaumont *et al.*, 1983; Mantione *et al.*, 1984) (see also the general remarks in § 1.3).

2.6.2 *The micromolar benzodiazepine binding site*

A third benzodiazepine binding site of rat brain membranes has been described by Bowling & DeLorenzo (1982) which binds several benzodiazepine derivatives with micromolar affinities in contrast to the nanomolar affinities of the central benzodiazepine receptor. The substrate specificity of these sites differs markedly from that of the central benzodiazepine receptor and does not mirror the pharmacological or clinical potency of the classical benzodiazepine derivatives. Bowling & DeLorenzo (1982) have proposed that affinity to this site might correlate with the potency of benzodiazepine to protect against electroshock, one of the few pharmacological properties of the benzodiazepines which does not correlate with binding to the central benzodiazepine receptor (Möhler & Okada, 1977). Although this hypothesis could explain observations about benzodiazepine derivatives inactive in the electroshock test but binding with high affinity to the benzodiazepine receptor (Haefely *et al.*, 1985), it should be mentioned that other authors have failed to find any evidence for micromolar benzodiazepine binding sites in rat brain membranes, even under the same experimental conditions as those used in the original report of Bowling & DeLorenzo (1982) (File *et al.*, 1984). On the other hand, DeLorenzo's group has recently replicated their original findings (Johansen *et al.*, 1985) and has reported comparable micromolar binding of [^{3}H]clonazepam to rat brain synaptosomal membranes and to neuronal membranes of the leech, the latter tissue being devoid of benzodiazepine receptors. Very interestingly, the same authors found that benzodiazepines in micromolar concentrations reversibly inhibit voltage-gated Ca^{2+} conductance in specific leech neurons in a dose-dependent manner and they conclude that benzodiazepines act as calcium channel blockers by interacting with the micromolar binding site. Their final conclusion, however, that the micromolar binding site might contribute to the therapeutic effects of the benzodiazepines (Johansen *et al.* 1985), gains little additional support from other available data, especially since benzodiazepine brain levels in the upper micromolar range are usually not obtained under therapeutic conditions.

2.6.3 *The indole and benzodiazepine binding site of human serum albumin*

Benzodiazepines bind with a high degree of specificity and even stereoselectivity to a single site of the human serum albumin molecule with partially very high affinities. Since the same single site mediates the stereospecific binding of tryptophan and related compounds, this site has been termed the 'indole and benzodiazepine binding site' (Müller & Wollert, 1979). This site is of considerable pharmacokinetic relevance, since it represents one of the two major drug binding sites of human serum albumin which are responsible for the interaction of nearly all drugs with the albumin molecule. The general properties of this site and their pharmacokinetic relevance for benzodiazepines and many other drugs have been summarized in several recent reviews (Müller & Wollert, 1979; Sellers *et al.*, 1983; Müller *et al.*, 1986*a*). This site is not involved in any of the pharmacological properties of the benzodiazepines, except that the plasma binding of these drugs contributes to their pharmacokinetics in man (Klotz, 1984). Thus, the indole and benzodiazepine binding site of human serum albumin clearly represents a silent receptor (see § 1.3) and represents an excellent example that specific and even stereospecific binding are not *per se* indicative of biological function.

2.7 Summary

The data summarized in this chapter clearly indicate the presence of highly specific benzodiazepine binding sites in all areas of the CNS, probably exclusively located on neurons. In terms of binding characteristics, e.g. saturability, substrate specificity, stereoselectivity, cellular as well as subcellular distribution and regional specificity, these sites exhibit clearly the properties typical for specific neuroreceptors present in the brain. However, binding specificity, although representing one of the important criteria of neuroreceptors, is not the only such criterion. This is best demonstrated by examples of several other specific benzodiazepine binding sites briefly reviewed in this chapter, e.g. the peripheral benzodiazepine binding sites, the micromolar benzodiazepine binding site and the indole and benzodiazepine binding site of human serum albumin, all of which are highly specific in terms of binding characteristics, but none of which is a functionally relevant receptor. Thus, in order to know that the brain-specific benzodiazepine binding sites represent the primary locus of benzodiazepine activity at the neuronal level and that the binding to these sites represents an essential step for the pharmacological activity of these drugs, more evidence than solely the presence of specific binding sites is needed.

3

The benzodiazepine receptor as the primary target of benzodiazepine drugs in the brain

As we learned at the end of the previous chapter, the presence of highly specific and even stereospecific binding sites of a given class of drugs in biological tissues cannot be considered final proof for the functional relevance of these sites. This is best demonstrated for the benzodiazepines by the examples of the pharmacologically inactive but highly specific (in terms of binding characteristics) peripheral benzodiazepine binding sites and the benzodiazepine binding site of human serum albumin (see § 2.6). Thus, in identifying a given population of specific binding sites as physiologically or pharmacologically relevant drug receptors or acceptors, several functional criteria must be fulfilled, and a clear correlation between binding and biological activity is most important. In the case of the benzodiazepine receptor, a variety of efforts has been made to demonstrate such functional criteria, which, on the whole, indicate clearly that the biological activity of benzodiazepines in man and other animals involves binding to this receptor system as the primary step within the molecular mechanism of action. These data will be reviewed in this chapter.

3.1 The relationship between receptor affinity and biological activity

3.1.1 *Correlations between* in vitro *affinity and pharmacological potency in animals*

As mentioned briefly in the previous chapter (see § 2.4), basic relationships between benzodiazepine receptor binding and pharmacological activity were reported in the first reports about the presence of specific benzodiazepine binding sites in the brain, inasmuch as pharmacologically inactive benzodiazepine derivatives or the inactive enantiomers of some benzodiazepine compounds exhibited very weak affinities for the benzodiazepine receptor. This approach has been extended by several authors to a variety of pharmacologically active benzodiazepine derivatives, all exhibiting different receptor affinities as well as different potencies in various pharmacological tests indicative for anticonvulsive, anxiolytic, muscle-relaxing and sedative properties. In most of these cases, very good correlations were found between *in vitro* receptor affinity and *in vivo* activity in animals, as can be seen from the relationship between receptor affinity and pharmacological activity as muscle relaxants in the cat (Fig. 3.1), which is taken from the first report of Möhler & Okada (1977) about the presence of benzodiazepine-specific binding sites in the rat brain. Similar good correlations have been reported between receptor affinity and pharmacological potency of the benzodiazepines for the

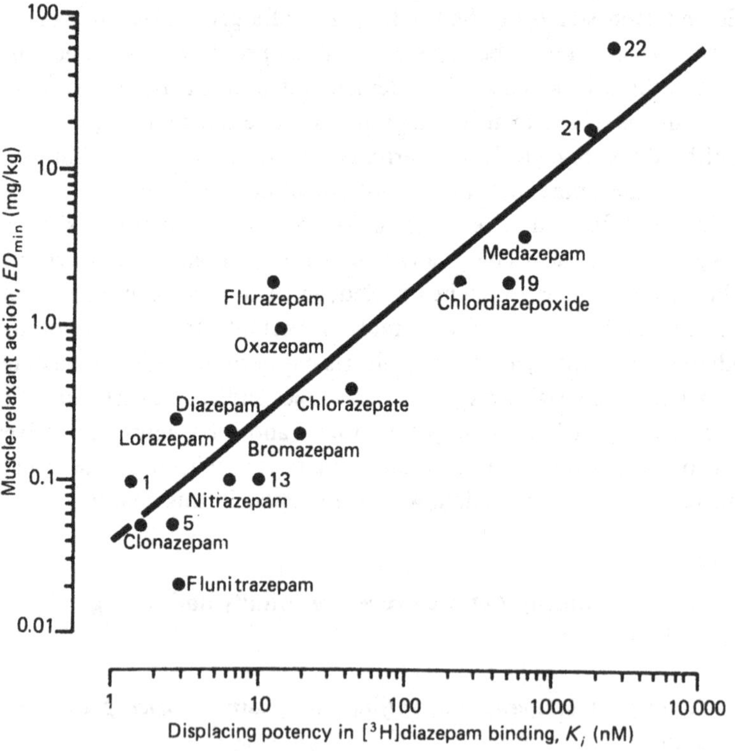

Fig. 3.1. The relationship between benzodiazepine receptor affinity *in vitro* as indicated by the inhibition constants (K_i, abscissa) and the pharmacological potency as muscle relaxants in cats as indicated by the minimum effective dose (ED_{min}, ordinate) of 17 different benzodiazepine derivatives ($r = 0.905, P < 0.001$). (Data are taken from Möhler & Okada, 1977, with permission.)

inhibition of electroshock-induced fighting in mice, antagonism against pentetrazol-induced convulsions in mice, the impairment of mouse rotarod performance, the performance of squirrel monkeys in a conditioned avoidance test, and the performance of rats in a continuous avoidance test (shock rate) (Möhler & Okada, 1977; Braestrup & Squires, 1978; Mackerer *et al.*, 1978; Speth *et al.*, 1980). However, some of these authors reported only weak correlations for the last test. On the other hand, all four groups found no or only weak correlations between *in vitro* receptor affinity and pharmacological potency in taming cynomolgus monkeys and in inhibiting electric shock-induced convulsions in mice. The possible significance of the micromolar benzodiazepine binding site for these pharmacological properties has already been discussed (§ 2.6.2). All these data show quite convincing correlations between receptor affinity and biological activity, especially if one considers that all these correlations neglect differences in the pharmacokinetics of the compounds. Thus, these data provide strong evidence that the binding to the benzodiazepine receptor is directly correlated with the pharmacological activity in animals.

3.1.2 *Correlations between* in vitro *affinity and therapeutic potency in man*

Similar attempts have been made to correlate *in vitro* receptor affinity with therapeutic potency of benzodiazepines in man. Figure 3.2 shows such a relationship between receptor affinity and the average hypnotic dose for adults, indicating again a very close correlation between affinity and potency. Similar correlations have been reported between benzodiazepine receptor affinity (with no difference if human or animal brain tissue is used) and the average therapeutic dose per day or the minimum effective antianxiety dose (Braestrup *et al.*, 1977; Braestrup & Squires, 1978; Möhler & Okada, 1978; Speth *et al.*, 1980). All these data clearly indicate a very good relationship between the therapeutic potency of benzodiazepines and their affinity for the benzodiazepine receptor, strongly suggesting that binding to the receptor is an important determinant for their activity in man. Thus, in simple terms receptor affinity represents the biochemical correlate to the therapeutic dose in man. It should be mentioned that there is no correlation between receptor affinity and the plasma half-life of the benzodiazepines in man (Table 2.4). Accordingly, the duration of the therapeutic effect of a benzodiazepine derivative shows no correlation at all with the receptor affinity. The explanation for these observations is given in Table 3.1, where the rate constants for association and dissociation and their respective half-lives are summarized. Even at low temperatures, association to and dissociation from the benzodiazepine receptor take place in minutes and are even faster at physiological temperatures. Thus, the amount of a given benzodiazepine derivative bound to the receptor can change very rapidly in response to the drug concentration in the brain. Since the latter is directly related to the overall

Table 3.1 *Rate constants of specific [^{3}H]flunitrazepam binding*

Half-lives of association and dissociation and the respective on- and off-rates of specific [^{3}H]flunitrazepam binding to rat brain homogenates at three different temperatures.

Temperature (°C)	$t_{1/2}$ association (s)	$t_{1/2}$ dissociation (s)	k_{+1} ($M^{-1}s^{-1}$)	k_{-1} (s^{-1})
0	834	942	7×10^5	7×10^{-4}
22	62	67	5×10^6	1×10^{-2}
35	12	11	1×10^7	6×10^{-2}

Source: Data are taken from Speth *et al.* (1978*b*).

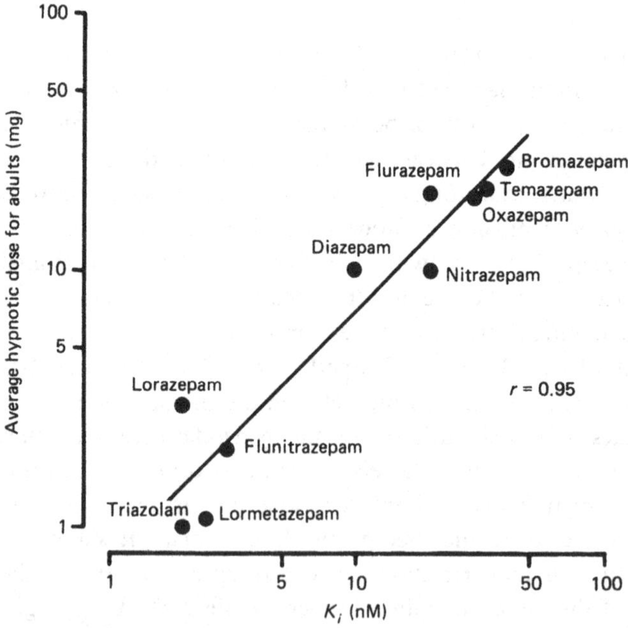

Fig. 3.2. The relationship between benzodiazepine receptor affinity *in vitro* as indicated by the inhibition constants (K_i, abscissa) and the therapeutical potency in man as indicated by the average hypnotic dose for adults (ordinate) of 10 different benzodiazepine derivatives used clinically as hypnotics. (Adapted from Müller, 1982*b*.)

elimination rate of the benzodiazepine derivative in the body (usually determined by the plasma half-life), receptor occupation and therefore the duration of the therapeutic effect in man are exclusively determined by the different pharmacokinetic parameters of the various benzodiazepine derivatives. In other words, benzodiazepines with very high as well as with low receptor affinities can have short as well as long plasma half-lives. At least for the benzodiazepine derivatives presently available (Table 2.4), there is no therapeutic advantage of high-affinity compounds over low-affinity compounds or vice versa.

Summarized in one sentence, out of the two parameters given in Table 2.4 for the commercially available benzodiazepine derivatives (in West Germany; not all are available in the United Kingdom), the receptor affinity determines the therapeutic dose while the elimination half-life mainly determines the duration of the therapeutic effect. (This simplification holds mainly for a single dose as it is given for the hypnotic use of the drugs. It should be quite clear that for multiple dosing, dose as well as elimination half-life are important to reach a given steady-state plasma level of the drugs.)

3.1.3 *Correlations between* in vivo *receptor affinity and biological potency*

As already mentioned, most of the correlations between receptor affinity *in vitro* and biological activity as summarized above did neglect differences of the pharmacokinetic properties of the drugs. If benzodiazepine derivatives with major differences in their pharmacokinetic properties are included, such correlations can become very poor. This is demonstrated by the example of the basically very good correlation between *in vitro* receptor affinity and average hypnotic dose for adults (Fig. 3.2), which has been plotted again using *in vitro* data from our laboratory (Fig. 3.3). As can be seen in Fig. 3.3*a*, a good correlation was found again for triazolam, diazepam, nitrazepam, temazepam and oxazepam. The two compounds midazolam and chlordiazepoxid, however, clearly did not fit into this correlation. Midazolam is much more potent at the receptor *in vitro*, as one would expect from its hypnotic dose, and the hypnotic dose of chlordiazepoxid is much smaller, as one would expect from its weak receptor affinity *in vitro*. Both findings can be explained easily on the basis of the pharmacokinetics of the drugs (Klotz, 1984). Midazolam is characterized by a pronounced first-pass metabolism, so that only 40–60% of the oral dose are systematically available. The reverse is the case with chloridazepoxid, which is metabolized to derivatives which are much more active than the parent compound (with respect to biological activity as

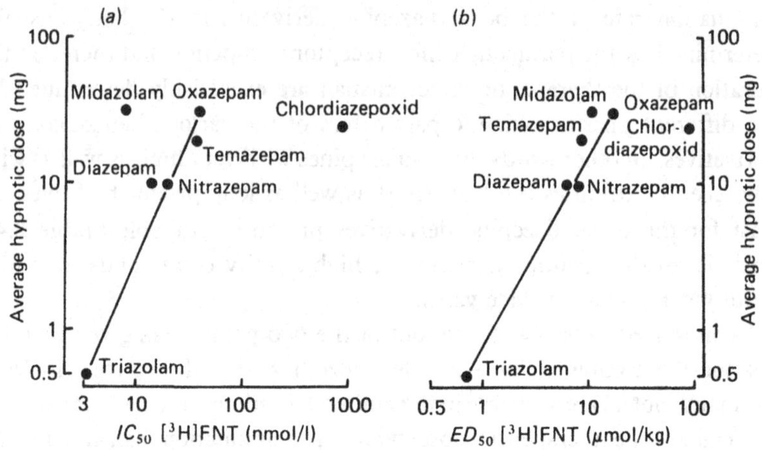

Fig. 3.3. The relationships between the average hypnotic dose in adults and (*a*) the *in vitro* benzodiazepine receptor affinity, as indicated by the inhibitory concentration 50% (IC_{50}) against specific [^{3}H]flunitrazepam binding to mouse brain homogenates or (*b*) the *in vivo* benzodiazepine receptor affinity, as indicated by the oral dose of the drugs which inhibits specific [^{3}H]flunitrazepam in the mouse brain *in vivo* by 50% (ED_{50}). For further experimental details see Müller & Stillbauer (1983).

well as to receptor affinity). Thus, for neither drug can *in vivo* receptor occupation be predicted from the *in vitro* receptor affinity. To overcome these problems, receptor affinity can also be determined *in vivo*. In this case it is usually given as ED_{50}, i.e. that *in vivo* dose which inhibits specific ligand binding *in vivo* by 50% by occupying 50% of the receptors present. If such *in vivo* data are used (Fig. 3.3*b*), the correlation between receptor binding and hypnotic activity becomes much better. The observation that chlordiazepoxid is still somewhat outside the correlation can be explained by differences in the metabolism of this drug between man and mouse.

If the same species is used for assaying *in vivo* receptor binding as well as biological activity, excellent correlations are found. One example is given in Fig. 3.4, which not only includes pharmacokinetically different but pharmacodynamically similar benzodiazepines like midazolam and chlordiazepoxid, but also some non-benzodiazepine agonists of the benzodiazepine receptor like zopiclone and Cl 218 872 (see § 2.4). These observations complete the conclusions made on the basis of correlations using *in vitro* receptor affinity and indicate clearly that, for a given species, a specific pharmacological effect is always elicited by doses of benzodiazepine receptor agonists which occupy the same fraction of the total receptor population in a given brain area. The observations also strongly suggest once again that binding to the benzodiazepine receptor

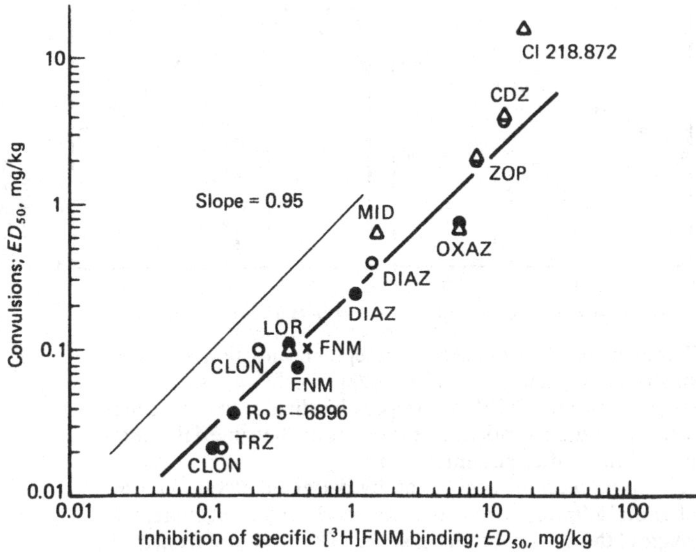

Fig. 3.4. The relationship between *in vivo* receptor binding (ED_{50} against specific [^{3}H]flunitrazepam binding, abscissa) and anticonvulsive potency (ED_{50} against pentetrazol-induced convulsions, ordinate) for several benzodiazepines and related drugs in mice. (Reproduced from Braestrup *et al.* (1983*b*) with permission.)

represents the primary step of the molecular mechanism of action of benzodiazepines and related compounds.

Accordingly, the determination of the fractional receptor occupancy over time represents an excellent pharmacokinetic parameter about the CNS kinetics of a given benzodiazepine derivative, taking into account the concentrations of the parent compound and its active metabolites at the locus of their pharmacological activity (brain). It is not surprising that this parameter correlates better with pharmacological activity than the determination of plasma or even brain levels of the drug investigated (Mennini & Garattini, 1983; Haefely, 1985). An example for the time course of receptor occupation by diazepam after a single oral dose is given in Fig. 3.5, where the very fast onset of receptor occupation even after oral administration is most remarkable.

3.2 Receptor occupation, spare receptors and pharmacological activity

As mentioned just now, correlations between *in vivo* receptor binding and pharmacological activity (see Fig. 3.4) clearly indicate the

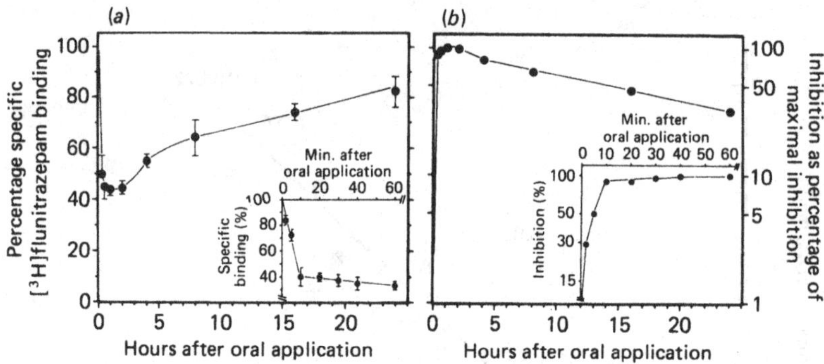

Fig. 3.5. Time course of benzodiazepine receptor occupation *in vivo* after oral administration of diazepam (7.5 μmol/kg) in the mouse.
(*a*) Inhibition of specific [^{3}H]flunitrazepam binding at various time intervals after oral administration. The inset shows the same data for the time from 2–60 min. after administration.
(*b*) Benzodiazepine receptor occupation by diazepam at various time intervals after oral administration. The data are the same but expressed as a percentage of the maximal effect observed. (Reproduced from Müller & Stillbauer, 1983.)

involvement of the benzodiazepine receptor in the pharmacological activity of these compounds. Moreover, such correlations strongly suggest three further conclusions.

1 Since the doses needed to elicit a given pharmacological response in 50% of the animals and the doses needed to inhibit specific binding to the receptor by 50% change from benzodiazepine to benzodiazepine always in a similar fashion, these effects are elicited by each of the drugs at a similar level of receptor occupation.
2 Since the pharmacological ED_{50} values are much lower than those for *in vivo* receptor binding, the pharmacological response (protection against pentretrazol-induced convulsions, Fig. 3.4) is already obtained by each of the drugs included in the correlation (Fig. 3.4) at a level of receptor occupation of about 25%, an observation which agrees with some earlier estimations (Duka *et al.*, 1979; Paul *et al.*, 1979).
3 Taking points 1 and 2 together, we can conclude that, at least for the anticonvulsive properties of the benzodiazepines, a large number of spare receptors is present and that the agonistic properties (intrinsic activity) of the drugs listed in Fig. 3.5 do not differ very much.

Similar correlations have also been reported for other pharmacological properties of the benzodiazepines: see the example presented in Fig. 3.6,

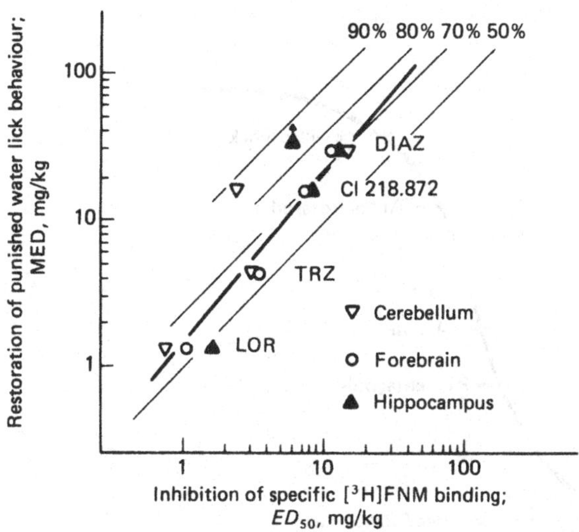

Fig. 3.6. The relationship between *in vivo* receptor binding (ED_{50} against specific [^{3}H]flunitrazepam binding, abscissa) and pharmacological activity in the water lick test (predictive for anxiolytic activity) (given as minimal effective doses, ordinate). Both parameters were determined in rats. The fine lines represent the theoretical curves indicating 50%, 70%, 80% and 90% receptor occupancy. (Modified from Braestrup *et al.*, 1983*b*.)

demonstrating the correlation between *in vivo* receptor binding and potency in the water lick test for anxiolytic activity in the rat. Very interestingly, since this pharmacological property is only observed at considerably higher doses of benzodiazepine derivatives, it can be concluded that anxiolytic activity needs a much higher level of receptor occupancy than anticonvulsive activity. From the data given in Fig. 3.6, it can be estimated that pharmacological activity in this test occurs at about 60–70% benzodiazepine receptor occupation. Although other data about receptor occupancy at anxiolytic benzodiazepine doses vary from study to study and from species to species, it is a consistent finding that receptor occupancy for anxiolytic effects is considerably higher than for anticonvulsive effects (Braestrup *et al.*, 1983*b*; Petersen *et al.*, 1986).

The correlation between receptor occupancy and pharmacological activity has recently been investigated in some detail by Petersen *et al.* (1986). These authors demonstrated that, in a given species, receptor occupancy is relatively low for pharmacological tests predictive of anticonvulsive activity, somewhat higher for tests predictive of anxiolytic activity, and considerably higher for tests predictive of muscle-relaxant activity (Fig. 3.7). Based on these and several other observations, the

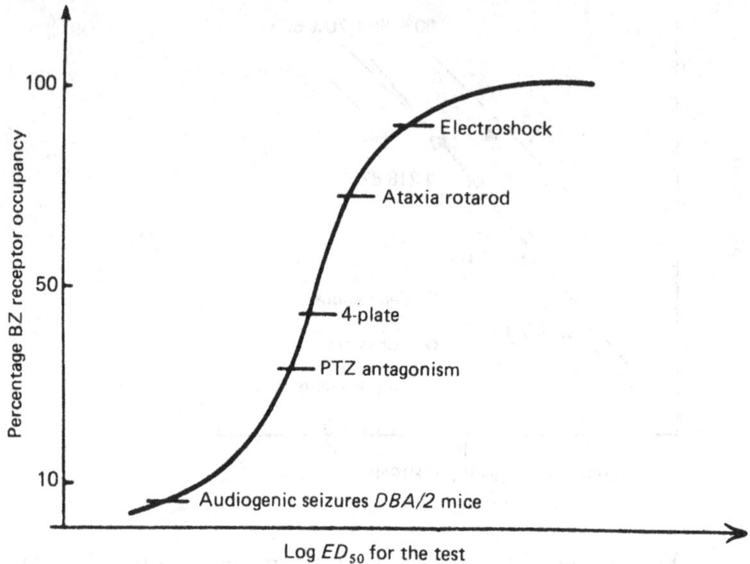

Fig. 3.7. The relationship between ED_{50} and benzodiazepine receptor occupancy in various tests in mice. The abscissa is arbitrary. Reproduced from Petersen *et al.* (1986).

The effectiveness of benzodiazepines against audiogenic and pentretrazol-induced convulsions is predictive for anticonvulsive properties, that in the 4-plate test for anxiolytic properties, and those in the ataxia rotarod and electroshock tests for muscle-relaxant properties.

still-speculative scheme in Table 3.2 can be given, indicating the relationship between different levels of receptor occupancy and the different pharmacological effects of the benzodiazepines. Conversely, with increasing levels of receptor occupancy needed to elicit a given pharmacological response, the number of spare receptors (the receptors which have to remain unoccupied) decreases. Thus, a major conclusion that can be drawn from all these findings is that the different doses of a given benzodiazepine derivative needed to elicit different pharmacological responses in experimental animals (for a review see Haefely *et al.*, 1981) can be explained by the different levels of receptor occupancy needed for these effects. Since receptor occupancy will be transduced to a receptor-mediated stimulus, it is clearly evident that some pharmacological properties of the benzodiazepines need more receptor-mediated stimuli than others.

No data are available concerning benzodiazepine receptor occupancy and clinical effects in man. However, since the general properties of the benzodiazepine receptor do not differ between animals and man (Chapter 5) and since we know from clinical experience that ataxia and muscle relaxation are usually seen only after high doses of benzodiazepines, it might be speculated that similar, but certainly not identical, correlations exist between receptor occupancy and clinical effects or side-effects in man.

3.3 Partial agonists of the benzodiazepine receptor

The very impressive correlations between *in vivo* benzodiazepine receptor occupancy and pharmacological response seen in many cases (see above) do not hold true for all benzodiazepine receptor agonists and all pharmacological properties of the benzodiazepines. This is shown by the data from our laboratory in Fig. 3.8. In agreement with the conclusions made above, all five benzodiazepine derivatives are more potent (having lower pharmacological ED_{50} values) in the pentetrazol test (anticonvulsive activity) than in the fighting mice test (anxiolytic activity). Both pharmacological properties correlate linearly with the ED_{50} for *in vivo* receptor binding. The two straight lines obtained from the correlations suggest that the two pharmacological properties are obtained at different levels of *in vivo* receptor occupation. The level, however, is similar for each of the five drugs in one single test. Similarly, muscle-relaxant properties (horizontal grid test) are observed for diazepam, clobazam, chlordiazepoxid and lofendazam at an even higher level of receptor occupation, which again is similar for the four drugs investigated. These data are compatible with the model presented in Fig. 3.7, indicating increasing but for each agonist similar fractional receptor occupation in relation to the different pharmacological properties. This model (Fig. 3.7), however, does not hold true for the 1,5-benzodiazepine arfendazam (Müller,

Table 3.2 *Benzodiazepine receptor occupancy and pharmacological response*

The relationship is shown between benzodiazepine receptor occupancy and the pharmacological (and clinical?) effects of a benzodiazepine derivative. Several of the effects may be overlapping.

Benzodiazepine receptor occupancy (Receptor-mediated stimulus)	Effects	Number of spare receptors
	Loss of consciousness Muscle relaxation Motor impairment Amnesia Hypnotic effect Antiepileptic effect Anxiolytic effect	

Source: According to Petersen *et al.* (1986).

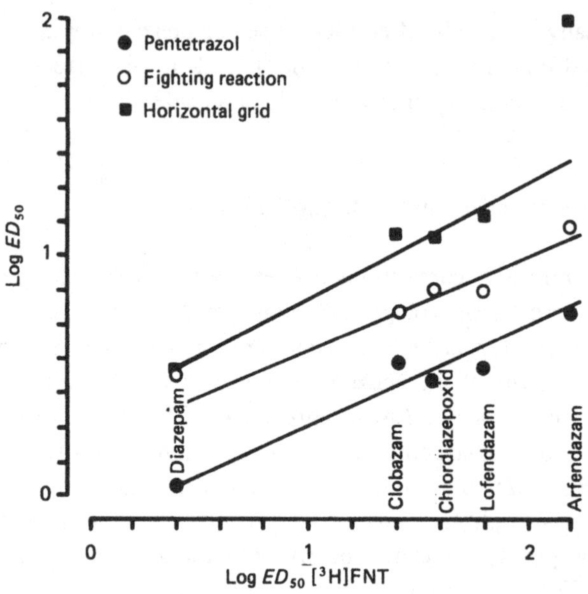

Fig. 3.8. The relationship between the potencies of five benzodiazepines as inhibitors of specific [^{3}H]flunitrazepam *in vivo* (whole mouse brain) as indicated by the ED_{50} [^{3}H]FNT (mg/kg, abscissa) and their potencies in three pharmacological tests in the mouse as indicated by the ED_{50} (mg/kg, ordinate). (Reproduced from Müller, 1985.)

1985), which exhibits muscle-relaxant properties only at much higher doses than one would expect from the correlation obtained for the other four benzodiazepine derivatives (Fig. 3.8), indicating that the muscle-relaxant properties of arfendazam are observed only at a considerably higher fractional receptor occupancy. Since studies with benzodiazepine receptor antagonists (see § 3.4) have clearly indicated that all three pharmacological properties of arfendazam are mediated by interaction with the benzodiazepine receptor, the classical explanation for the different properties of arfendazam is the assumption of a lower intrinsic activity of arfendazam relative to other benzodiazepines. In other words, arfendazam represents only a partial agonist of the benzodiazepine receptor.*

Similar pharmacological observations have been made for several other putative partial benzodiazepine receptor agonists (Haefely, 1984*b*; Stephens *et al.*, 1985), with the general tendency that the interval between the doses needed for anticonvulsive and anxiolytic effects or needed for sedative and

* Actually, arfendazam represents a prodrug. The active metabolite which is the true partial agonist of the benzodiazepine receptor is *N*-desmethylclobazam (Müller *et al.*, 1986*b*).

muscle-relaxant effects is much higher than for the classical benzodiazepine receptor agonists. Evidence for the presence of only partial agonistic properties at the benzodiazepine receptor can also be obtained from some biochemical *in vitro* assays (see § 4.1.4). Using these *in vitro* systems, most of the non-benzodiazepine agonists of the benzodiazepine receptor (see Fig. 2.8) seem to have lower intrinsic activities than the classical benzodiazepine derivatives. However, the differences are not very pronounced, especially if one compares these older partial agonists with some recently developed compounds (Haefely, 1984*b*; Stephens *et al.*, 1985; Petersen *et al.*, 1986). Thus, the pharmacological profiles of some of these drugs (Fig. 2.8) and of the classical benzodiazepines are not so much different. Our present knowledge would indicate that, with decreasing intrinsic (agonistic) activity, the interval between the anxiolytic and anticonvulsive doses on the one site and the sedative and muscle-relaxant doses on the other site becomes larger. This fits well the observations regarding the different levels of spare receptor present for the various pharmacological properties of benzodiazepine receptor agonists. For some of the newer compounds, intrinsic activity is so low than even very high doses, which will give 100% receptor occupation are not sufficient to produce muscle-relaxant effects in experimental animals (Haefely, 1984*b*). Experience with these compounds in man is very limited (Merz, 1984), but the idea of introducing such compounds as anxiolytics with less atactic and sedative side-effects than usually seen with classical benzodiazepines seems quite promising and might represent the most interesting approach to obtain benzodiazepine-related drugs with more selective therapeutic properties (see also § 9.1).

3.4 Benzodiazepine receptor antagonists

Certainly the most convincing approach to demonstrate a receptor-mediated effect of a given drug or biological compound (transmitter, hormone, modulator) is the blockade of this effect by specific and competitive antagonists. Classical examples of such more-or-less specific and competitive receptor antagonists are atropine in the case of the muscarinic cholinergic receptor, curare in the case of the nicotinic cholinergic receptor of the neuromuscular junction, and β-blockers in the case of the β-adrenergic receptor. Basically, the only pharmacological effect of such antagonists is their specific binding to a given receptor, which prevents the interaction of the agonist with the receptor and hence its biological effects. Since most of these antagonists inhibit the agonist binding competitively, very high agonist concentrations are able to overcome the receptor blockade by simply displacing the antagonist from the receptor or, better, its antagonist recognition site.

Very interestingly, more-or-less specific and competitive benzodiazepine receptor antagonists have been found during the last few years within several chemical classes of benzodiazepine receptor ligands including imidazabenzodiazepinones, phenylpyrazoloquinolines and β-carbolines. The chemical structures of some of these antagonists are shown in Fig. 3.9. All have in common a relatively high affinity for the benzodiazepine receptor, as indicated by the IC_{50} against specific [^{3}H]flunitrazepam binding values, which are in the low nanomolar range.

The prototype of these benzodiazepine receptor antagonists and certainly the most thoroughly investigated compound of this class of drugs is the imidazobenzodiazepinone Ro 15–1788 (Hunkeler *et al.*, 1981; Haefely, 1983; Haefely *et al.*, 1985). Ro 15–1788 is virtually devoid of any relevant intrinsic activity but potently antagonizes all relevant pharmacological effects of benzodiazepines as measured in biochemical, pharmacological or electrophysiological experiments. In binding experiments, Ro 15–1788 binds with high affinity and pronounced selectivity only to the

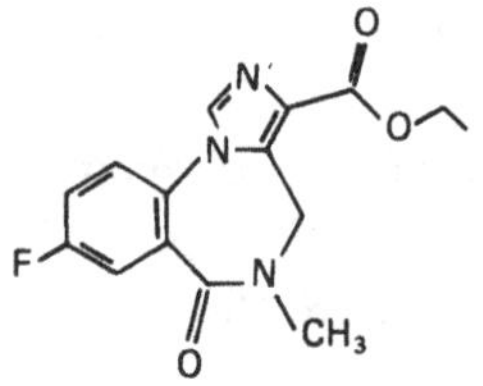

Ro 15–1788

(IC_{50} = 2.5)

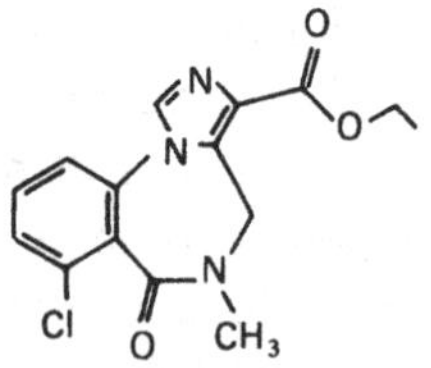

Ro 15–3505

(IC_{50} = 2.7)

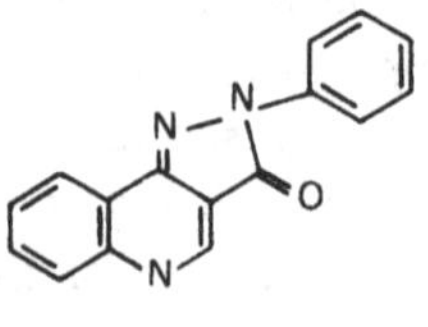

CGS 8216

(IC_{50} = 0.5)

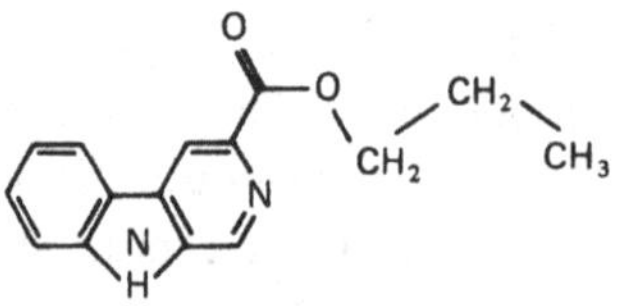

PrCC

(IC_{50} = 1.8)

Fig. 3.9. Structural formulae and benzodiazepine receptor affinity (given as IC_{50} value against specific [^{3}H]flunitrazepam binding in nmol/l) of four benzodiazepine receptor antagonists.

benzodiazepine receptor and represents one of the radioligands employed to label benzodiazepine receptors in direct binding experiments (see § 2.1). Similar binding characteristics (see Chapter 5) and pharmacological properties have been found for Ro 15–1788 in man, where this antagonist abolished practically all effects observed for benzodiazepine derivatives (Haefely, 1983).

In conclusion, the availability of highly selective and very specific benzodiazepine receptor antagonists has demonstrated definitely the significance of the benzodiazepine receptor as the primary target for benzodiazepines in the brain. It should be mentioned that the presence of competitive agonists and antagonists was the only evidence for the presence of all of our neurotransmitter receptors before the advent of direct binding techniques, which are only about 10 years old. Moreover, benzodiazepine receptor antagonists have become important research tools to elucidate many aspects of benzodiazepine receptor function: e.g. § 4.4 about the role of antagonists in investigating the function of the benzodiazepine receptor within the benzodiazepine receptor–GABA receptor–chloride channel complex, or § 6.2 about the role of antagonists in elucidating the possible physiological function of the putative endogenous ligand of the benzodiazepine receptor.

In general, other benzodiazepine receptor antagonists have properties similar to Ro 15–1788. They might differ in their intrinsic activity, which, although being generally very low, can be demonstrated in appropriate experiments (Haefely, 1983; Rodgers & Waters, 1985; File & Pellow, 1986).

4

The benzodiazepine receptor as a modulatory unit of GABAergic neurotransmission

Although GABA was only discovered as recently as in 1950, today we have convincing evidence that GABA represents the most important inhibitory neurotransmitter of the mammalian central nervous system. Estimates of the percentage of GABAergic synapses among all nerve endings range from 50% (forebrain) to about 30% for the whole mammalian central nervous system. These histological data are supported by iontophoretic studies indicating that nearly all central neurons can be affected by GABA (and therefore might possess GABA receptors). Thus, in quantitative terms, GABA probably represents the most important neurotransmitter of our brain (for reviews, see Snodgrass, 1983; Roberts, 1984).

The usual neuronal response of the activation of a GABA receptor is a hyperpolarizing IPSP (inhibitory postsynaptic potential) due to gating a chloride channel. Since some neurons have very high intracellular chloride concentrations, gating a chloride channel by GABA receptor activation may also explain depolarizing responses to GABA receptor agonists (e.g. primary afferent terminals in the spinal cord). Thus, the same neuronal mechanism can explain different effects on the membrane potential (Snodgrass, 1983; Simmonds, 1984; Haefely *et al.*, 1985).

Because of this broad functional role of GABA in the mammalian CNS, the early reports about a possible involvement of GABA in the mechanism of action of benzodiazepines were accepted very enthusiastically, since for the first time they provided a basis on which to combine the broad spectrum of pharmacological and therapeutic properties of the benzodiazepines with a specific neurotransmitter system. However, it took some time before the presumed GABA-mimetic properties of the benzodiazepines could be explained at the level of the GABAergic synapses of the CNS.

4.1 Functional evidence for GABA-mimetic properties of benzodiazepines

As already mentioned in the Introduction, the concept of benzodiazepines acting as GABA-mimetic drugs was introduced several years before the discovery of the benzodiazepine receptor. However, the possible mechanism of this GABA-mimetic activity was completely unknown, since benzodiazepines did not act via indirect mimetic mechanisms already known from other neurotransmitters, e.g. by enhancement of neuronal release, or by a blockade of the synaptic degradation of the neurotransmitter. Since the discovery of the benzodiazepine receptor, great progress has been made, and today we have a fairly clear picture of how benzodiazepines act as indirect GABA-mimetic agents and of the mechanisms by which benzodiazepines enhance inhibitory GABAergic transmission. Our present state of knowledge will be reviewed briefly in this chapter, but only to such an extent as to give a general understanding of this specific topic. For further details, the interested reader should refer to the reviews by Olsen (1981, 1982), Haefely *et al.*, (1983), Ticku (1983), and Tallman & Gallager (1985).

4.1.1 *Electrophysiology*

GABAergic inhibitory neurotransmission is mediated in the mammalian CNS by several kinds of GABAergic neurons and by two different types of neuronal response. If GABAergic neurons synapse presynaptically to axons of others neurons (axo-axonic synapses), GABA acts as a presynaptic inhibitory transmitter, probably by depolarizing the receptive axon (Fig. 4.1*a*). This kind of presynaptic inhibition has been found on the endings of primary afferents of spinal and cranial nerves (Fig. 4.2). All other kinds of GABAergic synapses are axo-somatic or axo-dendritic, where the GABAergic neurons might be small interneurons (collateral inhibition or recurrent inhibition, Fig. 4.1b_1, b_2) or projecting principal neurons (Fig. 4.1*c*). The GABAergic synapses in this second group mediate so-called postsynaptic inhibition and account for the majority of GABAergic synapses in the CNS (Simmonds, 1984). Interestingly, both kinds of GABAergic inhibition (pre- as well as post-synaptic) are mediated by the same $GABA_A$ receptor subtype, which operates by gating a chloride channel of the neuronal membrane. The electrophysiological response, however, is different in the case of presynaptic inhibition (depolarization) from that in the case of postsynaptic

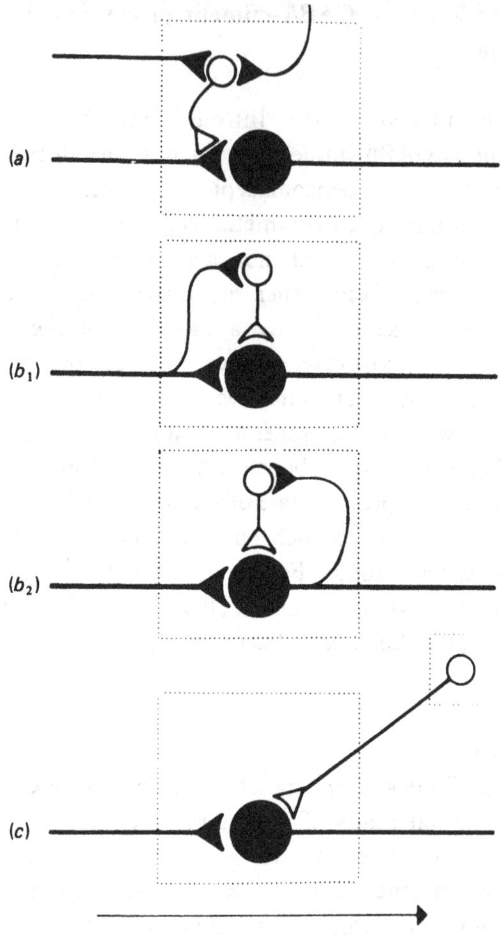

Fig. 4.1. Schematic diagrams of inhibitory GABAergic circuits: (*a*) Presynaptic inhibition by axo-axonic synapse, (b_1) postsynaptic inhibition, collateral inhibition, (b_2) postsynaptic inhibition, recurrent inhibition, and (*c*) postsynaptic inhibition by a projecting neuron. GABAergic neurons are depicted in white, excitatory neurons in black. (Reproduced from Haefely, 1980.)

inhibition (hyperpolarization) due to the different intracellular chloride concentrations of the receptive neurons (Simmonds, 1984; Snodgrass, 1983). However, in most cases of GABA-mediated responses in the mammalian CNS, benzodiazepines have been shown to enhance the effects of GABA in spite of its pre- or post-synaptic locus of action. Some schematic diagrams of neuronal circuits containing inhibitory GABAergic neurons are summarized in Fig. 4.2. In all these cases, benzodiazepines have been

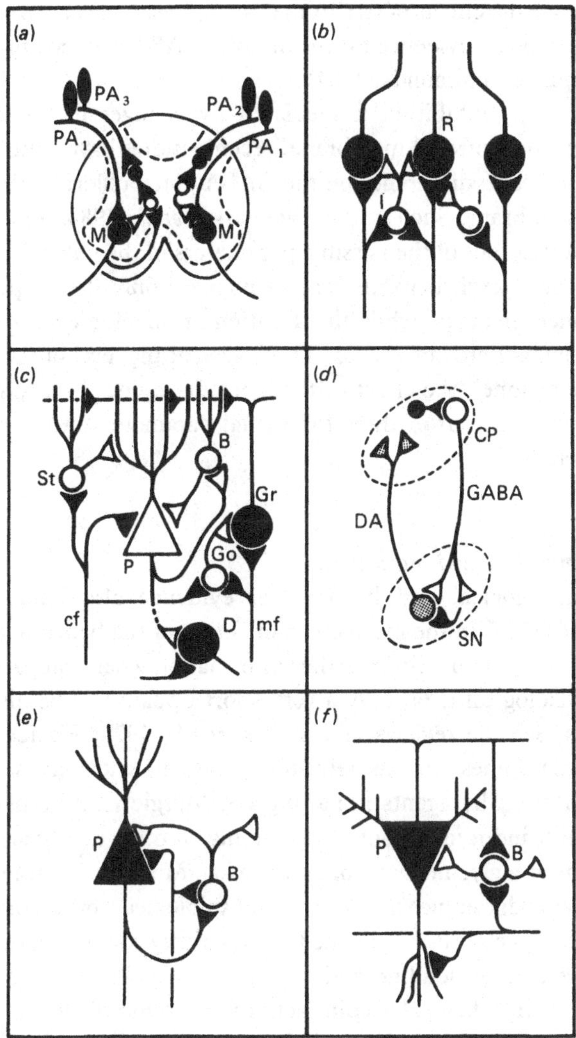

Fig. 4.2. Schematic diagrams of the main neuronal circuits containing GABAergic synapses, where benzodiazepines have been found to enhance transmission. GABAergic neurons are shown in white, excitatory neurons in black. (*a*) Spinal cord (M, motorneuron; PA, primary afferents), (*b*) dorsal column nuclei (R, relay cell; I, interneuron), (*c*) cerebellar cortex (P, Purkinje cell; Gr, granule cell; Go, Golgi cell; B, basket cell; St, stellate cell; D, output neuron of Deiters' nucleus; cf, climbing fibre; mf, mossy fibre), (*d*) neostriatum and substantia nigra (CP, caudate-putamen; SN, substantia nigra; DA, nigrostriatal dopamine pathway; GABA, GABAergic striatonigral pathway), (*e*) cerebral cortex (P, pyramidal cell; B, basket cell), (*f*) hippocampus (P, pyramidal cell, B, basket cell). (Reproduced from Haefely, 1984*a*.)

shown to enhance the effects of GABA in electrophysiological experiments, giving very convincing evidence for the indirect GABA-mimetic properties of benzodiazepines (Simmonds, 1984).

Since GABAergic inhibition is mediated by changes in the chloride conductance of the neuronal membrane, recent studies have concentrated on the effects of benzodiazepines on the GABA-gated chloride channel of the neuronal membrane. Such studies (see Barker *et al.*, 1984, for a review) have indicated that, out of the possible parameters of the chloride channel at the microscopic level, benzodiazepines increase only the frequency of chloride channel openings, while the duration of opening events and the channel conductance are not altered. Thus, even at the level of the GABA-gated chloride channel, the effect of the benzodiazepines is very specific, inasmuch as only one out of three functional parameters of the chloride channel is altered.

4.1.2 *Pharmacology and biochemistry*

Pharmacological and biochemical evidence also points to an involvement of GABA in the mechanism of action of the benzodiazepines. Since these data contribute little further information when compared with the electrophysiological data, only a very short update will be given (for further details, see the reviews of Schallek *et al.*, 1979; Haefely *et al.*, 1981). Benzodiazepines are usually more potent antagonists against convulsions induced by agents impairing GABAergic neurotransmission than against those induced by convulsants acting via other neuronal systems (e.g. strychnine as a glycine receptor antagonist). Moreover, a large variety of effects of benzodiazepines at the electrophysiological, biochemical and pharmacological levels can be blocked by relatively low doses of GABA antagonists such as bicuculline and picrotoxin. Finally, in a variety of experimental settings, benzodiazepine activity is profoundly lowered when the brain levels of GABA are reduced by inhibitors of GABA synthesis. All these data suggest indirect GABA-mimetic properties of the benzodiazepines, albeit without indicating the possible mechanism of action.

4.1.3 *Histochemistry*

The hypothesis of a GABA-mimetic activity of the benzodiazepines was strongly supported by histological data indicating that the presence of the benzodiazepine receptor in all brain regions was strongly correlated with the presence of GABAergic nerve terminals. One of the first reports on this subject came from Placheta & Karobath (1979) who found a comparable regional distribution of GABA receptors and benzodiazepine receptors, with the consistent finding of more GABA receptors than benzodiazepine receptors in all brain regions studied. A more direct approach involves the combination of the benzodiazepine receptor autoradiographic technique with immunohistochemical methods for glutamic acid decarboxylase, the marker enzyme of GABAergic neurons (Möhler & Richards, 1983; Kuhar, 1983). Using such methods, strong evidence for the coexistence of benzodiazepine receptors with GABAergic synapses was demonstrated at the light microscopic as well as electron microscopic level. Final evidence for the co-localization of the benzodiazepine receptor and the GABA receptor came from the recent data about the isolation and purification of a synaptic macromolecule containing both the benzodiazepine and the GABA receptor (Schoch *et al.*, 1984; Häring *et al.*, 1985). In conclusion, strong evidence exists that most if not all benzodiazepine receptors are co-localized with GABA receptors. Up to now, little evidence has been obtained for the presence of benzodiazepine receptors not biochemically linked to GABA receptors. On the other hand, since the CNS in man contains many more GABA receptors than benzodiazepine receptors, it is generally assumed that the majority of GABA receptors are not linked to benzodiazepine receptors (Bowery *et al.*, 1984).

The GABA receptors associated with the benzodiazepine receptors are always of the $GABA_A$ subclass, which can be specifically antagonized by bicuculline. No evidence exists that $GABA_B$ receptors (which can be specifically activated by the drug baclofen) are associated with benzodiazepine receptors (Bowery *et al.*, 1984). The low-affinity binding component of the $GABA_A$ receptor is usually assumed to be connected to the benzodiazepine receptor (Bowery *et al.*, 1984), but this assumption is still in dispute.

4.1.4 *Receptor interactions: effects of GABA receptor agonists on benzodiazepine receptor binding and vice versa*

Strong evidence for a close functional relationship between the GABA receptor and the benzodiazepine receptor also comes from binding experiments (see Braestrup *et al.*, 1983*a*, for a review). When brain membranes are washed very thoroughly or are treated in some other ways to remove all endogenously present GABA, the affinity of benzodiazepines and other benzodiazepine receptor agonists for the benzodiazepine receptor can be increased by the *in vitro* addition of GABA or other GABA receptor agonists. Such a simple experiment is shown in Fig. 4.3. In other words, activation of the GABA receptor by agonists increases agonist binding to the benzodiazepine receptor, strongly suggesting allosteric interactions between the two receptors. This effect, usually called GABA shift or GABA ratio, is very specific for benzodiazepine receptor agonists and is not observed for antagonists of the benzodiazepine receptor. Accordingly, the GABA ratio represents not only an important argument for a functional interaction between both receptors, but also the best *in vitro* test system

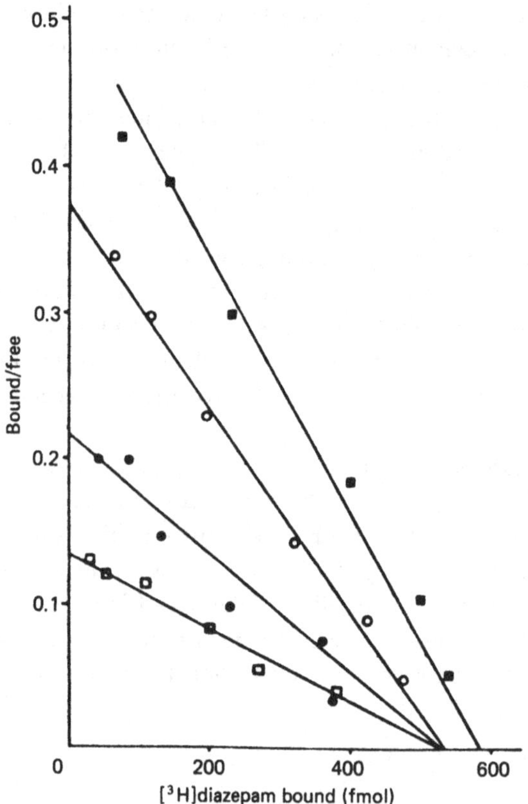

Fig. 4.3. The effect of GABA receptor agonists on the binding of (^{3}H]diazepam to thoroughly washed rat brain membranes. • = control binding; ○ = binding in the presence of GABA 10 μmol/l; ■ = binding in the presence of muscimol, a GABA receptor agonist, 10 μmol/l; □ = binding in the presence of (+) bicuculline methiodide 100 μmol/l, a GABA receptor antagonist. The binding data are presented as a Scatchard plot (see Fig. 2.5). The similar intercepts of the straight lines with the abscissa indicate that GABA receptor ligands change only the binding affinity and not the number of benzodiazepine receptors. (Reproduced from Tallman *et al.*, 1978.)

for differentiating benzodiazepine receptor agonists, antagonists and inverse agonists (see § 4.4). However, the GABA shift cannot explain the GABA-mimetic properties of the benzodiazepines.

It is interesting that an increase of the affinity of agonist binding to the GABA receptor in the presence of benzodiazepines has also been described (Johnston & Skerritt, 1984). This effect could explain much better the GABA-mimetic properties of benzodiazepines. However, it is not the final explanation, since the potency of benzodiazepine receptor agonists to enhance GABA receptor binding does not correlate at all with their pharmacological potency or their affinity for the benzodiazepine receptor. Thus, although both phenomena strongly indicate close functional interactions between the receptors, they do not represent the biochemical correlate of the GABA-mimetic properties of benzodiazepines.

4.2 The GABA receptor–benzodiazepine receptor–chloride channel complex

Taking together all the evidence (see § 4.1.1 to 4.1.4), the following model of the GABA receptor–benzodiazepine receptor unit of the GABAergic synapse can be given (Fig. 4.4). Although several parts of this

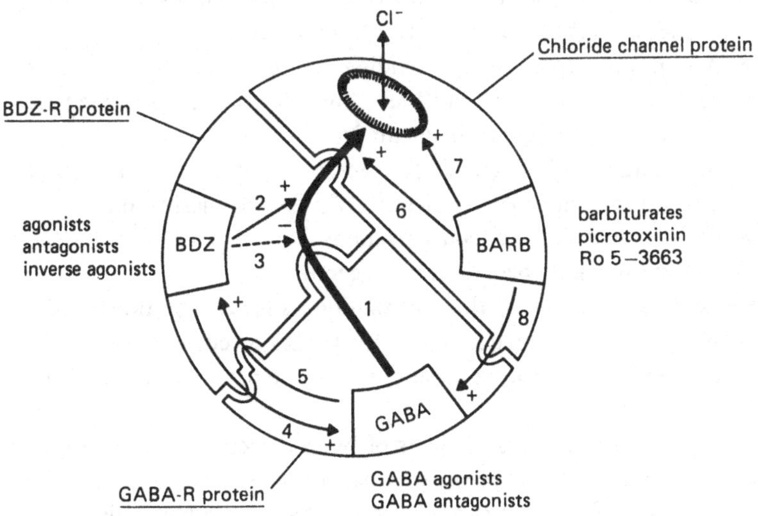

Fig. 4.4. Hypothetical model of GABA receptor–benzodiazepine receptor–chloride channel complex of the GABAergic synapse. For explanation of numbers 1 to 8 see text. (Reproduced from Polc *et al.*, 1981.)

model have been confirmed in biochemical experiments, others are still based exclusively on functional data.

This model assumes the presence of a multifunctional macromolecular unit, consisting of the chloride channel, the GABA receptor, the benzodiazepine receptor and a third recognition site binding drugs like barbiturates as agonists and some convulsants like picrotoxin as antagonists. All four units can interact with each other, finally resulting in a very complicated pattern of responses.

1 Activation of the GABA receptor by an agonist leads to a conductance change of the chloride channel, as we have already seen (§ 4.1.1). Although this represents the physiologically most important part of the model, the biochemical mechanism of the GABA-induced gating of the chloride channel is not yet known.
2 Agonist binding to the benzodiazepine receptor enhances the effect of GABA agonists on the chloride channel by increasing the frequency of channel opening events. Again, the biochemical mechanism is not yet known.
3 Binding of inverse agonists (see § 4.4) to the benzodiazepine receptor has the opposite effect, i.e. it decreases the frequency of channel opening events.
4 Agonist binding to the benzodiazepine receptor enhances agonist affinity at the GABA receptor.
5 Agonist binding to the GABA receptor enhances agonist binding to the benzodiazepine receptor (GABA ratio).
6 Agonists at the picrotoxin binding site (e.g. barbiturates) at low concentrations also enhance the GABA-receptor-mediated activation of the chloride channel.
7 Barbiturates at high (possibly anaesthetic) concentrations seem to activate the chloride channel directly (hyperpolarization).
8 Barbiturates at low concentrations can also enhance agonist binding to the benzodiazepine receptor.

The effects of agonists at all three recognition sites can be prevented by specific antagonists, e.g. bicuculline at the GABA receptor, Ro 15–1788 at the benzodiazepine receptor, and picrotoxin at the barbiturate recognition site.

This model summarizes the effects of benzodiazepines on GABAergic neurotransmission. It also explains why barbiturates at low concentrations have a pharmacological spectrum similar to that of the benzodiazepines, but given at high (anaesthetic) concentration can produce a much more pronounced depression of the CNS due to their direct effects on the chloride conductance (hyperpolarization) of the neuronal membrane.

Today, it can be assumed that a variety of other convulsive or anticonvulsive drugs also interact with one or several of the different parts of this multifunctional complex. For further details, see the reviews of Olsen (1981, 1982) and Ticku (1983).

4.3 The chain of events from benzodiazepine receptor occupation to pharmacological response

As we learnt above, benzodiazepines increase the frequency of chloride channel opening events under the influence of GABA after interacting with the benzodiazepine receptor as part of a large multifunctional unit. Although this basic mechanism is understood fairly well, it is very hard to imagine how this effect at the level of the neuronal membrane is transformed into the very specific pharmacological and therapeutic properties of the benzodiazepines. Moreover, if we consider the broad role of GABA as inhibitory transmitter in the CNS, how is it that enhancing the synaptic effects of this rather unspecific inhibitory neurotransmitter by benzodiazepines or related benzodiazepine receptor agonists results in such specific pharmacological properties of these drugs? No definite answer is available for either question, since not all of the steps starting with the conductance change of the neuronal membrane up to the pharmacological effect are yet understood clearly. On the other hand, since many of these steps are known, an interim model can be given (Figs. 4.5 and 4.6), explaining the mechanism of action of the benzodiazepines, starting with the conductance change of the neuronal membrane and leading up to the final pharmacological effect. This model also summarizes most of our knowledge about the mechanism of action of the benzodiazepines, although it is important to stress again that several aspects of it are still hypothetical.

Benzodiazepines modulate the GABA-operated chloride channel within the benzodiazepine receptor–GABA receptor complex (Fig. 4.5, right). This complex is part of the postsynaptic neuron (Fig. 4.5, left) at a GABAergic inhibitory synapse. Similar GABAergic synapses can be found in many areas of the CNS, since many neurons receive inhibitory GABAergic input (Fig. 4.6). In a given brain region, one type of neuron might be more sensitive than others for the enhanced GABAergic inhibition, which probably explains the specificity of the benzodiazepine effects. Best evidence for this assumption is available for the anxiolytic activity of the benzodiazepines, where an enhanced inhibition on serotoninergic target neurons in the limbic system might be relatively

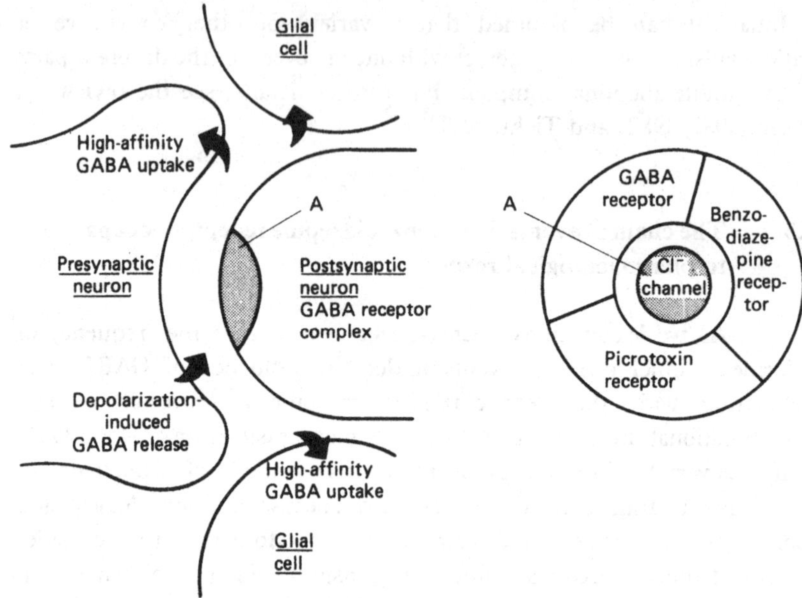

Fig. 4.5. Schematic presentation of the pre- and post-synaptic part of a GABAergic synapse (left). Part A, the GABA receptor–benzodiazepine receptor–chloride channel complex, is given again (right) on a larger scale (see also Fig. 4.4). (Modified from Müller, 1982*b*.)

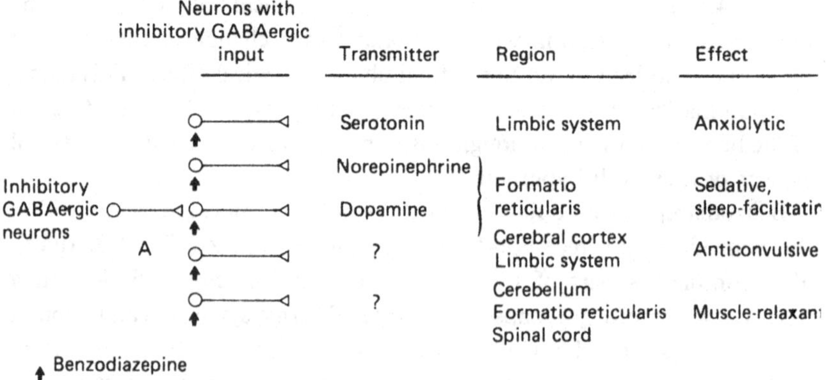

Fig. 4.6. Hypothetical model to explain the postsynaptic enhancement of GABAergic inhibition by benzodiazepines in several brain regions and its possible relationship to pharmacological effects. Part A, the GABAergic synapse with the benzodiazepine receptor, has been shown in Fig. 4.5 on a larger scale. (Modified from Müller, 1982*b*.)

important (Fig. 4.6). Speculations about brain regions and target neurons involved in the other pharmacological properties of the benzodiazepines are also given in Fig. 4.6.

The question which remains is why some neurons or neuron systems of a given brain region are significantly affected by benzodiazepines and others not. It seems unlikely that this can be explained by the presence or absence of benzodiazepine receptors or GABAergic synapses, since both are widely distributed in most brain areas. A possible explanation might be the relatively small overall effect of benzodiazepines on neuronal activity, since the intensity of the potentiating action of benzodiazepines on GABAergic inhibition is rather small and results in only a small shift of the GABA dose–response curve without altering the intensity of the maximum effect of GABA (Haefely, 1984*a*) (see Fig. 4.7). Obviously, benzodiazepines are most active around the middle part of the dose–response curve of GABA alone, while much less pronounced effects can

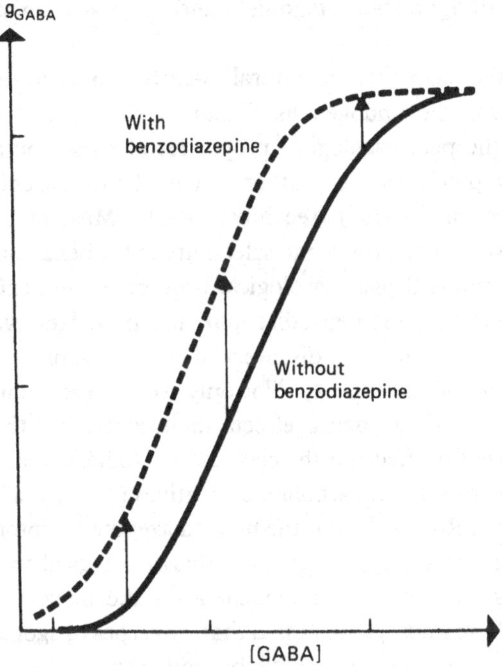

Fig. 4.7. Schematic diagram to show the possible effect of a benzodiazepine on the dose–response curve of GABA. The relative enhancement of GABAergic activity depends on the synaptic GABA concentration and accordingly on the activity of the GABAergic neuron, as indicated by the arrows. g_{GABA} means the conductance change induced by GABA. (Reproduced from Haefely, 1984*a*.)

be expected when the GABAergic activity alone is very high or very low (see the arrows in Fig. 4.7). In other words, the maximum effect of benzodiazepines on GABAergic inhibition is not only rather small, but also is seen within only a narrow range of GABAergic activity. Both effects might contribute to the highly specific pharmacological properties of the benzodiazepines, since even in the same brain region the relatively small enhancement of GABAergic inhibition by benzodiazepines might be sufficient to alter the activity of only one type of neuron. Thus, the assumption that benzodiazepines act specifically in our brain by enhancing the synaptic function of the rather unspecific inhibitory neurotransmitter GABA is not contradictory, but represents a very plausible concept to explain the mechanism of action of this important class of psychotropic drugs.

4.4 Benzodiazepine receptor ligands with different intrinsic activity: the concept of agonists, antagonists and inverse agonists

Soon after the discovery of several β-carboline derivatives as putative candidates for the endogenous ligand of the benzodiazepine receptor, studies on the pharmacological properties of these compounds indicated benzodiazepine-opposite rather than benzodiazepine-like properties (convulsive, anxiogenic) (see Nutt, 1983). Most of these β-carbolines bind with very high affinity and selectivity to the benzodiazepine receptor. Thus, their unusual pharmacological properties were explained by antagonistic properties at the benzodiazepine receptor. However, this assumption had to be revised after the discovery of benzodiazepine receptor antagonists like Ro 15–1788 (see § 3.4). Not only were these compounds virtually without any pharmacological effects themselves, but they also were able to antagonize the effects of the classical benzodiazepines as well as the opposite effects of some β-carboline derivatives (Nutt, 1983). Due to the high selectivity of Ro 15–1788 for the benzodiazepine receptor, these observations supported the assumption that the pharmacological properties of these β-carbolines (see above) are mediated via the benzodiazepine receptor. Moreover, these findings suggested that two types of agonist exist for the benzodiazepine receptor, one with benzodiazepine-like and one with benzodiazepine-opposite properties, and that the effects of both types of agonist can be blocked by Ro 15–1788, acting as a rather classical receptor antagonist. This concept, unusual as it is in pharmacology, has received more and more experimental support during the last few years. (Braestrup *et al.*, 1983*a*; Möhler & Richards, 1983; Haefely, 1984*a*; Tallman & Gallager, 1985).

These data are summarized in the scheme given in Fig. 4.8 about the different types of benzodiazepine receptor ligands. This basically indicates the existence of a continuum of agonistic properties, ranging from full agonists (benzodiazepines) on the one site to inverse agonists (or contragonists) (DMCM) on the other site. As already mentioned in § 3.3, the spectrum of benzodiazepine receptor agonists ranges from full agonists (full intrinsic activity) to several groups of partial agonists of reduced intrinsic activity (Fig. 4.8). At the end-point of the agonist spectrum are the antagonists like Ro 15–1788, which are nearly, but not completely, devoid of agonistic properties (intrinsic activity).

Very interestingly, other benzodiazepine receptor antagonists like ECC and FG 7142 are also not completely devoid of intrinsic activity, but show slight proconvulsive and anxiogenic properties, indicating the switch from agonists (benzodiazepine-like) to inverse agonists already within the group of benzodiazepine receptor antagonists. As we have seen for the agonists, the spectrum of inverse agonists ranges from antagonists with slight inverse

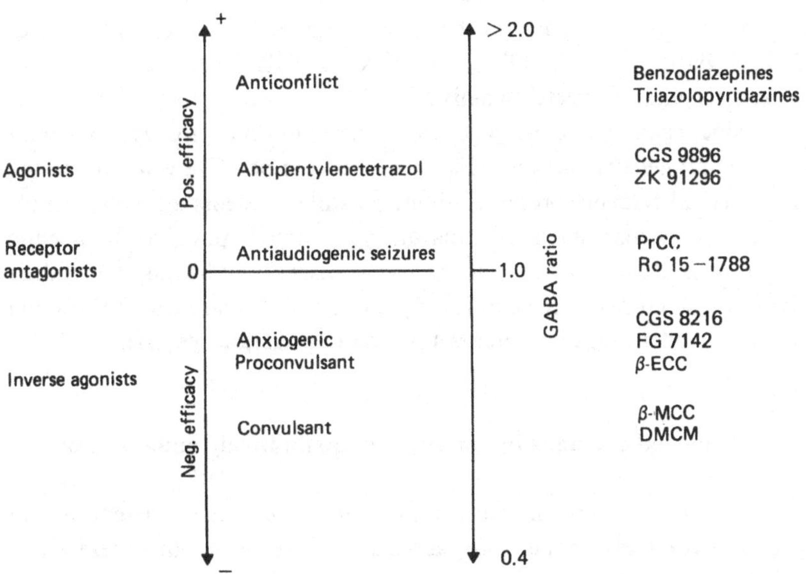

Fig. 4.8. The continuum of agonistic properties of benzodiazepine receptor ligands ranging from positive to negative efficacy in relation to the pharmacological properties and to the GABA ratio as a biochemical *in vitro* test predictive of the different intrinsic activities. (Adapted from Braestrup *et al.*, 1983*a*.)

intrinsic activity (or negative efficacy) over partial inverse agonists (MCC) to more or less full inverse agonists (DMCM), where the latter compounds are potent convulsants comparable to pentetrazol (Braestrup *et al.*, 1982).

Comparable to the benzodiazepine receptor agonists, where the presence of GABA increases the benzodiazepine receptor affinity with increasing agonistic properties (positive efficacy) (Fig. 4.8), the affinity of inverse agonists for the benzodiazepine receptor is decreased by GABA with increasing inverse agonistic properties (negative efficacy) (Fig. 4.8) (Braestrup & Nielsen, 1981). Accordingly, the GABA ratio (IC_{50} in the absence of GABA over the IC_{50} in the presence of GABA, see § 4.1.4) can be used as an *in vitro* test for positive as well as negative efficacy of benzodiazepine receptor ligands (Braestrup *et al.*, 1983*a*). Again, the GABA effects on benzodiazepine receptor affinity do not explain the inverse agonistic properties, but only seem to parallel these effects, since inverse agonists decrease GABAergic inhibition by interacting with the benzodiazepine receptor. As is the case with the enhancement of GABAergic inhibition by benzodiazepine receptor agonists, the biochemical mechanism of the decrease of GABAergic transmission by inverse agonists is not yet understood. However, the final effect of the inverse agonists is a decrease of the frequency of the chloride channel opening events under GABA (Barker *et al.*, 1984), an effect exactly opposite to that of benzodiazepines or related agonists.

In conclusion, the concept of benzodiazepine receptor agonists with positive and negative efficacy (Fig. 4.8) seems to be quite valid due to the experimental evidence present, although it still represents the only example for such a mechanism in pharmacology. Although possible therapeutic uses of benzodiazepine receptor inverse agonists might be few, if any, their discovery has contributed significantly to our understanding of the function of the benzodiazepine receptor within the GABAergic synapse.

4.5 Benzodiazepines in current use: qualitatively equal or not?

The discussion of whether the benzodiazepines in current use are qualitatively equal or not is nearly as old as the benzodiazepines themselves, but it still represents an important controversy between clinicians and pharmacologists or clinical pharmacologists. Many clinicians feel that there are qualitative differences, e.g. one compound might be more activating while another might be more sedative. Moreover, it has been proposed to classify the classical benzodiazepine derivatives in terms of their relative anxiolytic sedative, anticonvulsive and muscle-relaxant potencies (Laux,

1982). However, all these attempts to differentiate the benzodiazepines qualitatively are subjective opinions rather than the results of objective experimental studies. While there is general agreement that, in a daily routine, differences can be found between benzodiazepines, these are usually explained by differences in the pharmacokinetics (mainly onset and duration of action) and by the fact that in many cases the recommended doses of the commercially available benzodiazepines are not equipotent. However, it is clear from my many discussions with clinicians that this explanation is not accepted by all of them, although it represents the opinion of most clinical pharmacologists.

It is quite conceivable that the major developments made in recent years with respect to the molecular mechanism of action of the benzodiazepines should be able to clarify this important controversy further. To translate the question for equal properties in pharmacological terms, we have to look for similar or dissimilar efficacies or intrinsic activities, or we have to ask if all clinically used benzodiazepines are full agonists of the benzodiazepine receptor.

In relation to both questions, two major conclusions can be made. First, good evidence exists that no major differences in the intrinsic activities are present between the presently available benzodiazepines. This is clearly demonstrated by the excellent correlations between receptor occupation and specific pharmacological effects (as discussed in § 3.2). Secondly, whether small differences in efficacy exist is still open to question. Recent data from Chan & Farb (1985) suggest that some benzodiazepines in clinical use differ qualitatively in potentiating the GABA-induced conductance change of spinal cord neurons (Fig. 4.9). However, whether these differences in efficacy at the level of the neuronal membrane are of any relevance for the claimed differences between the therapeutic properties of some benzodiazepine derivatives remains to be demonstrated.

4.6 Summary

Overwhelming evidence indicates today that benzodiazepines act by enhancing the synaptic effects of the inhibitory neurotransmitter GABA. Although the mechanism of this GABA-mimetic effect is not yet understood in every detail, many aspects of the mechanism are already known fairly well.

What remains to be determined is whether all properties of the benzodiazepines are mediated by GABA. At present, little is known about GABA-independent effects of benzodiazepines, at least with respect to

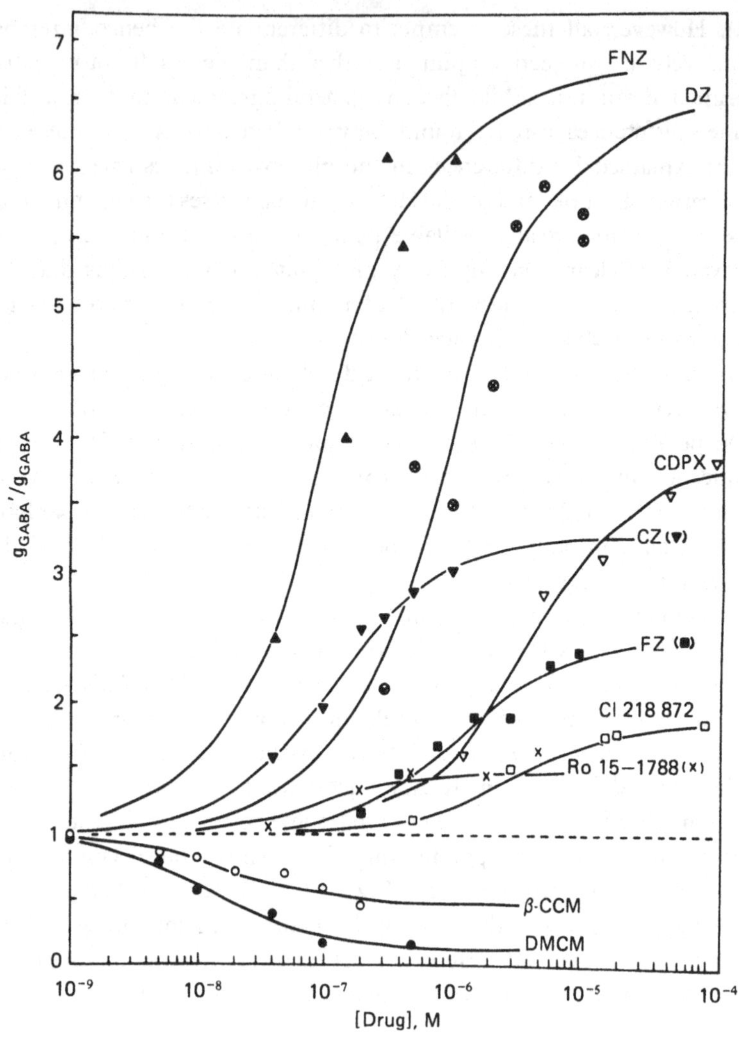

Fig. 4.9. Concentration–response curves for the potentiation or reduction of the GABA-induced conductance change of mouse spinal cord neurons by benzodiazepine receptor agonists, antagonists and inverse agonists. g_{GABA} and g_{GABA}' represent the conductance changes induced by the same concentration of GABA without and in the presence of the benzodiazepine derivative, respectively. It is interesting that the maximal potentiation of GABA response for several classical benzodiazepines differs significantly, indicating different efficacies or intrinsic activities. FNZ = flunitrazepam, DZ = diazepam, CDPX = chlordiazepoxid, CZ = clonazepam, FZ = flurazepam, β-CCM = β-MCC. (Reproduced from Chan & Farb, 1985, with permission.)

their therapeutic properties. It is outside the scope of the present book to review these GABA-independent effects, e.g. effects on adenosine uptake, on calcium transport and calcium conductance, and on phospholipid methylation. The interested reader should refer to the review by Haefely *et al.* (1985). GABA-independent mechanisms also involve the peripheral benzodiazepine binding site (see § 2.6.1) and the micromolar benzodiazepine binding site (see § 2.6.2), whose putative functions have already been discussed. Thus, while GABA-independent effects of benzodiazepines can presently not be ruled out completely, they are certainly without major relevance for the therapeutic effects of the benzodiazepines.

5

The benzodiazepine receptor in human brain

Soon after the discovery of benzodiazepine receptors in the brains of rats and other experimental animals, several reports were published about the presence of this receptor system in the human brain (Braestrup *et al.*, 1977; Möhler & Okada, 1978; Speth *et al.*, 1978*a*). In general, few differences between the benzodiazepine receptor systems in human and animal brain were found in these and several subsequent studies.

5.1 General properties

In terms of binding constants and average densities, no major differences are present between benzodiazepine receptors in animal and human brains. This is supported by the data of Sieghart *et al.* (1985), who recently compared the affinity and density of benzodiazepine receptors in human and rat cortex membranes using two different radioligands (Table 5.1). As indicated by these data, no differences in ligand affinity and only small differences in maximal binding capacity were found between human and rat cortex. Moreover, when the substrate specificities of the benzodiazepine receptor in human and animal brain were compared using the inhibition constants of a variety of benzodiazepines or related compounds for specific radioligand binding, very similar K_i values were usually found. This is nicely demonstrated by the data shown in Fig. 5.1, indicating a very close correlation between the IC_{50} values (inhibitory concentration 50%) against specific [^{3}H]FNT binding of a large variety of benzodiazepine receptor agonists, antagonists and inverse agonists in three areas of rat and human brain. Similar findings have been reported by Möhler & Okada (1978). Moreover, the same authors showed that the

Table 5.1 *Radioligand binding to benzodiazepine receptors on cortical membranes of man and rat*

Data for dissociation constants (K_D) and maximal number of binding sites (B_{max}) are calculated by Scatchard analysis of saturation curves.

Ligand	Species	K_D (nmol/l)	B_{max} (pmol/mg prot.)
$[^3H]$FNT	Man	2.7 ± 0.5	2.2 ± 0.1
	Rat	2.3 ± 0.1	2.8 ± 0.1*
$[^3H]$Ro 15–1788	Man	1.2 ± 0.1	2.3 ± 0.1
	Rat	1.5 ± 0.1	2.9 ± 0.1*

Note:
*Significantly different, $P < 0.01$

Source: Data are taken from Sieghart *et al.*, (1985).

stereospecificity of the benzodiazepine receptor is similar in human and in rat brain membranes.

5.2 Regional distribution

Few important differences between the regional distribution of the benzodiazepine receptor in human and animal brain have been found.

As in all other vertebrate species investigated, the benzodiazepine receptor is widely but unevenly distributed within the human CNS, with little evidence for its presence on peripheral organs. Its regional distribution in the human CNS, as determined in two studies using *post mortem* brain samples (Table 5.2), mirrors fairly well the regional distribution found in the CNS of other species (§ 2.2.2), with high densities in the cortex, hippocampus and cerebellum, and low densities in the medulla and the spinal cord. This fairly similar regional distribution does not mean, however, that no species differences are present, although the differences that have been observed are only seen for small and specific brain areas rather than for whole brain regions (Young & Kuhar, 1979).

Similar to findings in experimental animals, benzodiazepine receptors have been demonstrated outside the brain in the human spinal cord (Young & Kuhar, 1979), in the human retina (Borbe *et al.*, 1982), and in the

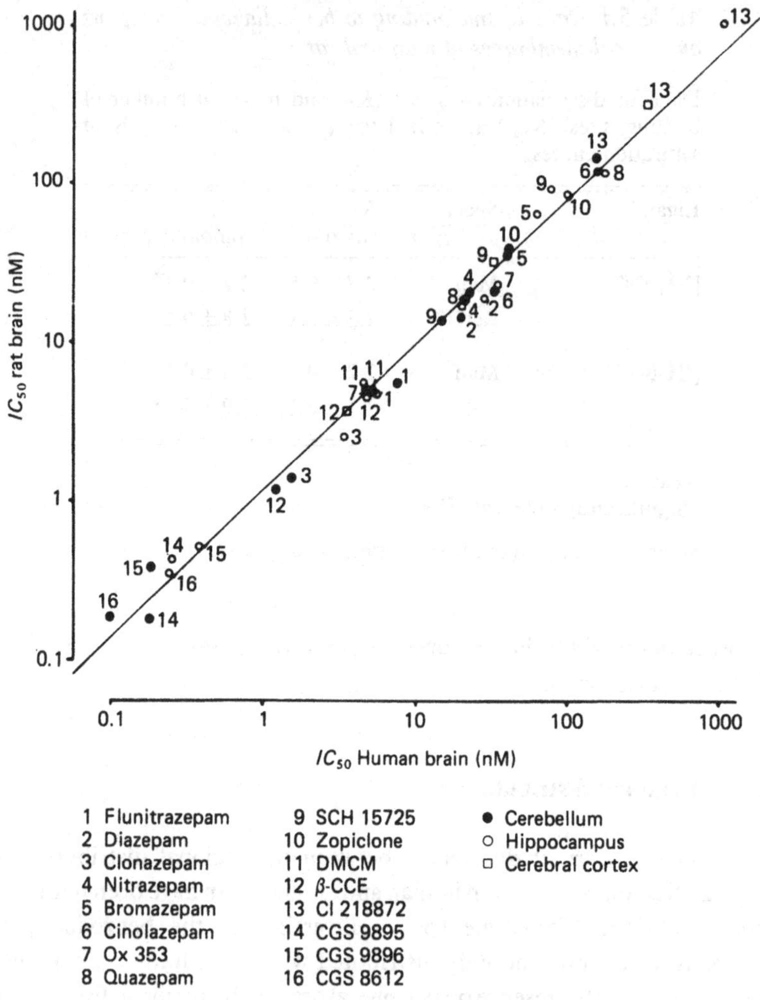

Fig. 5.1. Correlation between the IC_{50} values of a large variety of benzodiazepine receptor ligands in three regions of rat or human brain. (β-CEE = β-ECC.) (Reproduced from Sieghart *et al.*, 1985.)

human pineal gland (Lowenstein *et al.*, 1984). Their presence in the human pituitary is questionable (Grandison *et al.*, 1982; Voigt *et al.*, 1984).

5.3 Receptor subclasses

Using direct binding techniques as well as autoradiographic methods, benzodiazepine receptor subclasses of the BZ_1 and BZ_2 subtypes have also been identified in human brain (Niehoff & Whitehouse, 1983; Chiu *et al.*, 1984; Montaldo *et al.*, 1984). However, in the relative distribution of both subclasses, some distinct differences have been found between human and animal brain. The percentage of BZ_2 receptors in the human cerebellum is much higher than that found for most animal species (Montaldo *et al.*, 1984) and differences in the relative distribution of both subclasses between man and rat have also been described for some areas

Table 5.2 *Regional distribution in human brain*

Properties of specific [^{3}H]diazepam binding in *post mortem* human brain samples B_{max} = maximal number of sites, as determined from Scatchard plots, K_D = dissociation constant.

Brain region	B_{max}	(pmol/mg prot.)	K_D	(nmol/1)
Frontal lobe cortex	0.86	1.2*	3.5	7.0*
Temporal lobe cortex	0.67	1.2*	4.9	7.5*
Occipital lobe cortex	0.84	1.1*	4.8	7.0*
Cerebellar cortex	0.58	0.73*	4.2	5.8*
Vermis	0.76	0.72*	5.7	8.0*
Hippocampus	0.67	0.61*	4.2	6.5*
Amygdala	0.51	0.72*	9.0	6.7*
Hypothalamus	0.45	0.52*	7.4	8.2*
Nucleus accumbens	—	0.43*	—	6.5*
Thalamus	0.33	0.41*	4.6	8.7*
Nucleus caudatus	0.44	0.38*	4.3	8.5*
Putamen	0.36	0.36	4.1	6.8*
Globus pallidus	0.36	0.30*	4.1	6.2*
Nucleus dentatus	0.16	0.16*	7.0	8.7*
Substantia nigra	—	0.29*	—	10.6*
Tegmentum	—	0.18*	—	10.1*
Olive	—	0.16*	—	14.1*
Corpus callosum	0.11	0.05*	20.0	6.4*
Pons	0.16	0.16*	5.0	14.2*
Medulla oblongata	0.20	0.15*	12.0	21.9*
Medulla spinalis	0.21	—	7.0	—

Note:
*Data are from Möhler & Okada (1978).

Source: All other data are from Braestrup *et al.*, (1977).

of the hippocampus (Niehoff & Whitehouse, 1983; Manchon *et al.*, 1985). The functional relevance of these findings, however, is not yet known.

At the molecular level, the heterogeneity of benzodiazepine receptor proteins seems to be larger in human than in animal (rat) brain (Sieghart *et al.*, 1985), but the final relevance of these findings for the small but distinct differences in the regional distribution of the two subclasses remains to be demonstrated.

5.4 The benzodiazepine receptor–GABA receptor complex

A variety of data indicate that in human as in animal brain the benzodiazepine receptor represents part of a large supramolecular structure consisting of the benzodiazepine receptor, the GABA receptor, the picrotoxin binding site and the chloride channel (see Chapter 4). Evidence for this assumption comes from data about the stimulation of benzodiazepine receptor binding by GABAergic agonists in human brain (Reisine *et al.*, 1980*a*; Sieghart *et al.*, 1985) and by several agonists of the picrotoxin binding site (Sieghart *et al.*, 1985). Moreover, the regional distribution of the benzodiazepine receptor in human brain, as determined by receptor autoradiography, is fairly similar to the regional distribution of immunoreactivity against monoclonal antibodies raised in the mouse against the whole solubilized benzodiazepine receptor–GABA receptor complex from bovine brain (Schoch *et al.*, 1985). These data suggest that in human as in animal brain the benzodiazepine receptor is part of a similar supramolecular complex and that the biochemical characteristics of this complex are similar in human and animal brain.

5.5 Ontogenetic development

Benzodiazepine receptor binding has been detected in human fetal brain (cortex or whole brain preparations) between weeks 12 and 15 of pregnancy. The affinity was similar to that of adult human brain, but the maximal density was only about 10% of the adult levels (Aaltonen *et al.*, 1983). When compared with similar studies in fetal brains of mice or rats (Braestrup & Nielsen, 1978; Regan *et al.*, 1980), where benzodiazepine receptor levels are between 5 and 10% of the adult level at mid-gestation, their development in human fetal brain might show some, but obviously not major, differences. Data about the postnatal development of benzodiazepine receptors in human brain are not known. Their level at birth amounts to about 35% and 23% of the adult level in the rat and mouse brain respectively and reaches the adult level within 3 to 4 weeks after birth (Braestrup & Nielsen, 1978; Regan *et al.*, 1980).

5.6 Peripheral benzodiazepine binding sites

A few reports indicate the presence of peripheral-type benzodiazepine binding sites in human brain, with some evidence for a lower density when compared with the density of experimental animals (Schoemaker *et al.*, 1982; Owen *et al*, 1983). The density of these sites is slightly elevated in the frontal cortex of Alzheimer patients (Owen *et al.*, 1983) and in the putamen of patients who died of Huntington's chorea (Schoemaker *et al.*, 1982), but is unchanged in the frontal cortex of patients who died of dialysis encephalopathy (Kish *et al.*, 1985*b*) (see Table 5.3). Since peripheral benzodiazepine binding sites in the CNS might occur preferentially on glial cells, their increased levels in the brains of some patients have been interpreted as a sign of gliosis (Owen *et al.*, 1983).

Peripheral benzodiazepine binding sites have also been described on human pituitary cells (Voigt *et al.*, 1984), on human lymphocytes (Moingeon *et al.*, 1983), and on human platelets (Bénavidès *et al.*, 1984*b*).

Table 5.3 *Pathological changes of peripheral benzodiazepine binding sites in human brain*

Changes are given as significant changes of the specific binding of [^{3}H]Ro 5–4864 in relation to human brain samples of patients without neurological or psychiatric disorders.

Disease	Brain region	% change of specific [^{3}H]Ro 5–4864 binding	Reference
Senile dementia, Alzheimer type	Temporal cortex	+28	Owen *et al.* (1983)
Chorea Huntington	Nucleus caudatus	± 0	Schoemaker
	Globus pallidus	± 0	*et al.* (1982)
	Putamen	+51	
Dialysis encephalopathy	Frontal cortex	± 0	Kish *et al.* (1985*b*)

As in the animal brain, the pharmacological as well as the putative physiological relevance of these sites in human brain tissue is unclear.

5.7 *In vivo* labelling by positron emission tomography

Using ^{11}C-labelled flunitrazepam or ^{11}C-labelled Ro 15–1788, benzodiazepine receptors have been visualized by positron emission tomography in the human brain *in vivo* (Mazière *et al.*, 1981; Persson *et al.*, 1985; Samson *et al.*, 1985), using similar techniques to those introduced in animal experiments (Comar *et al.*, 1979; Ehrin *et al.*, 1984; Hantraye *et al.*, 1984). Using this technique, specific binding of the radioligand could be demonstrated in human brain with highest density in the medial occipital cortex, followed by the cerebellum, frontal cerebral cortex, thalamus and pons (Persson *et al.*, 1985; Samson *et al.*, 1985), which correlates fairly well with the data obtained from post-mortem homogenate studies (see § 5.2). Although the positron emission tomography method

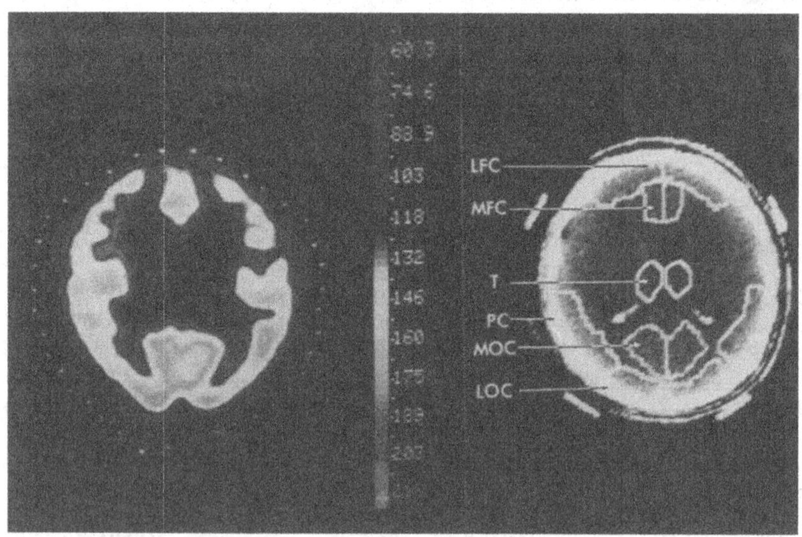

Fig. 5.2. PET and CT scans from the same section through the brain of a 43-year-old man. *Left*: PET scan showing benzodiazepine receptor binding of [^{11}C]Ro 15–1788. The scale indicates the relationship between colour and density. *Right*: CT scan showing some regions of interest used for quantification of radioactivity. LFC = lateral frontal cortex, MFC = medial frontal cortex, T = thalamus, PC = parietal cortex, MOC = medial occipital cortex, LOC = lateral occipital cortex. (Reproduced from Persson *et al.*, 1985.)

still has a limited spatial resolution, it might become the method of choice for future studies on the properties of the benzodiazepine receptor in human brain *in vivo*, as it has also been suggested for the *in vivo* visualization of several other receptor systems (Mintrun *et al.*, 1984; Phelps & Mazziotta, 1985). A few preliminary data about *in vivo* benzodiazepine receptor visualization in psychiatric patients have already been published (see § 7.3.1). An example of brain imaging of benzodiazepine receptors in man by positron emission tomography is given in Fig. 5.2.

5.8 Summary

A large variety of experimental evidence indicates that the benzodiazepine receptor in human brain exhibits all the general characteristics found for this system in the brain of experimental animals. Accordingly, most of the data about the molecular and biochemical properties of the benzodiazepine receptor in animal brain can probably be extrapolated to human brain as well. This, however, does not imply that all functional data about benzodiazepines can be extrapolated from animals to man as well. Even if the same brain region possesses the same density of benzodiazepine receptors, the functional relevance of these receptors might differ considerably from animals to man or even from one animal species to another. Thus, functional data obtained in animals can only be used to interpret benzodiazepine effects in man if a correlation between the effect in the experimental animal and a specific effect in man has been proven.

6

Is there a physiological function?

The major problem related to the benzodiazepine receptor centres around the questions of whether this system possesses a physiological function, or even if such a physiological function has to be assumed at all. This controversy has already been mentioned in the Introduction (§ 1.3). One side argues that, since the benzodiazepine receptor represents only a postsynaptic subunit of the GABAergic synapse allosterically modulating the activation of chloride channels by GABA, there is no reason to postulate a specific and independent role of its own for the benzodiazepine receptor system and the benzodiazepine receptor might represent only a drug acceptor site. However, as little final evidence exists for the general presence of such 'drug acceptors' as highly specific drug recognition sites without a physiological function, the arguments of the other side in favour of a putative endogenous role become more and more convincing. Thus, it seems rather unlikely that this system was developed during evolution at the step from non-vertebrates to vertebrates by mere coincidence and remained unchanged over the whole evolution of all vertebrates without our brain having any use for it. It is also rather unlikely that this highly specific receptor was developed by evolution for the sake of some large drug companies in the twentieth century making good profits by selling ligands for this system!

The most likely explanation for the presence of benzodiazepine receptors in our brain would therefore be the presence of an endogenous 'benzodiazepine-like' ligand for these binding sites. Unfortunately, such a compound has not yet been identified unequivocally. On the other hand, a variety of evidence for its presence in our brain is presently coming from three major aspects of benzodiazepine receptor research (Table 6.1), e.g. directly from experiments dedicated to the identification of the putative ligand itself and indirectly from studies in animals and man about pharmacological properties of 'pure' benzodiazepine receptor antagonists indicative of the presence of such a compound. Indirect evidence also comes from observations about benzodiazepine receptor sub- or super-sensitivity, phenomena usually assessed for physiologically relevant receptor systems. All three aspects will be reviewed here.

6.1 The search for the endogenous ligand

As discussed above, the finding that the benzodiazepine receptor must be activated by the binding of specific ligands in order to function as a modulatory subunit of the GABA receptor implies that its putative physiological function must be connected with the presence of an endogenous ligand. Accordingly, many attempts have been made to identify this putative endogenous benzodiazepine-like compound, and these will be reviewed in this section. Previous reviews on the same topic but on a much less comprehensive scale have been given by Müller (1981*a*, 1982*a*), Hamon & Soubré (1983) and by Davis *et al.* (1984).

6.1.1 *General strategies*

Several different approaches have been employed by laboratories all over the world to identify a compound with biological activity mediated through the benzodiazepine receptor (Table 6.2). In all cases, one has to be aware that the biological activity of this putative compound could be benzodiazepine-like or opposite to the effects of benzodiazepines. In pharmacological terms, the putative ligand could be a benzodiazepine receptor agonist or an inverse benzodiazepine receptor agonist (see § 4.4). Alternatively, the presence of more than one endogenous effector can be assumed with pharmacological properties from agonist to inverse agonist, modulating the gain at which the major or primary transmitter GABA works over a fairly large range (Davis *et al*.. 1984). From this uncertainty

Table 6.1 *The search for the endogenous ligand: areas of research giving direct or indirect evidence for its presence*

1	Direct identification of a putative endogenous ligand
2	Pharmacological studies using benzodiazepine receptor antagonists indicative of the presence of an endogenous ligand
3	Experimental findings about sub- or super-sensitivity and other measures of receptor plasticity

about the possible biological activity of the putative ligand, the question emerges about which pharmacological tests should be used to test for these compounds, which could be anticonvulsive or convulsive, anxiogenic or anxiolytic, and stimulating or sedative. Accordingly, for all the approaches outlined in Table 6.2, biological activity is usually determined first in benzodiazepine receptor binding assays and secondly in animal models indicative for anticonvulsive and convulsive or indicative for anxiolytic anxiogenic properties. Thus, the pharmacological properties of the many candidates for the putative ligand are not identical, but all will inhibit benzodiazepine receptor binding *in vitro* (Table 6.2).

6.1.2 *Active compounds isolated from biological materials*

The most direct approach for the demonstration of an endogenous effector of the benzodiazepine receptor would be its isolation and chemical identification from biological materials like brain extracts, liquor or urine (Table 6.2). In this respect, several chemically and biologically unrelated compounds have been isolated (Table 6.3). Their properties and their current status as possible endogenous ligands can be summarized as follows.

Nicotinamide

Nicotinamide has been isolated from acetone extracts of rat and bovine brain as one of three benzodiazepine receptor-binding inhibiting compounds (Möhler *et al.*, 1979). Like the two other compounds (inosine and hypoxanthine), nicotinamide has a very low affinity for the benzodiazepine receptor with an IC_{50} of about 4 mmol/l (Möhler *et al.*, 1979). But unlike the two other compounds also present in acetone extracts, nicotinamide showed benzodiazepine-like biological activities in several

Table 6.2 *The search for the endogenous ligand: general strategies and experimental approaches employed*

1 Isolation of active* compounds from biological materials, e.g. urine, liquor, and brain homogenates
2 Screening of already known biological compounds for possible activity*
3 Synthesis of active* biological model compounds (biomimetic approach)

Note:
*Active means binding to the benzodiazepine receptor and/or biological activity similar to agonists or inverse agonists.

electrophysiological and neuropharmacological experiments predictive for anxiolytic, anticonvulsive, muscle-relaxant and hypnotic activity (Möhler *et al.*, 1979). However, other investigators could not confirm a benzodiazepine-like biological activity of nicotinamide in various neuropharmacological experiments (Slater & Longman, 1979; Lapin, 1981; Petersen & Lassen, 1981). In agreement with these *in vivo* findings, the affinity of nicotinamide for the benzodiazepine receptor *in vitro* is not increased by the presence of GABA (the best *in vitro* test for benzodiazepine-like agonistic activity, see § 4.1.4). Moreover, the effects of nicotinamide on neuronal activity cannot be antagonized by the benzodiazepine receptor antagonist Ro 15–1788 (Bold *et al.*, 1985), further pointing against benzodiazepine receptor-mediated agonistic properties (Morgan & Stone, 1983). Probably the most important arguments against a role for nicotinamide as an endogenous ligand are the quite low brain concentrations of this compound of about 0.1 μmol/g (Möhler *et al.*, 1979), which, together with the IC_{50} of 4 mmol/l, make an *in vivo* receptor occupation by nicotinamide very unlikely. Furthermore, nothing is known about the presence of an endogenous system regulating the brain concentration of nicotinamide in terms of neuronal release and re-uptake, two mechanisms which one would expect to be present for a co-transmitter or neuromodulator.

Table 6.3 *The search for the endogenous ligand: putative candidates*

1 Active* compounds isolated from biological materials:
- Nicotinamide
- Inosine and hypoxanthine
- Ethyl β-carboline-3-carboxylate
- Tribulin
- Nephentin
- Several not yet identified peptides or proteins
- Diazepam displacing activity in human CSF
- Diazepam binding inhibitor (DBI)

2 Active* compounds present in the CNS, but not directly isolated from biological materials:
- Thromboxane A_2
- Prostaglandin A_1 and A_2
- Thyroxine
- Harmane and norharmane
- Melatonin and *N*-acetyl-5-methoxy-kynurenamine

Note:
*Active means binding to the benzodiazepine receptor and/or biological activity similar to agonists or inverse agonists.

In conclusion, little firm evidence suggests a physiological function for nicotinamide at the benzodiazepine receptor.

Inosine and hypoxanthine

Like nicotinamide, both inosine and hypoxanthine have been identified as active, e.g. benzodiazepine receptor-binding inhibiting components of brain extracts from rat and bovine brain (Skolnick *et al.*, 1978*a*, 1980; Asano & Spector, 1979; Möhler *et al.*, 1979). Also like nicotinamide, the affinities of both compounds for the benzodiazepine receptor are very low with IC_{50}s of about 1 mmol/l (Skolnick *et al.*, 1978*a*; Asano & Spector, 1979). Both purines, but especially inosine, have been thoroughly investigated for benzodiazepine-like pharmacological properties. The results are equivocal, since agonistic but also antagonistic properties have been reported. For example, inosine is effective against pentetrazole- and caffeine-induced convulsions (Skolnick *et al.*, 1979; Marangos *et al.*, 1981*b*) and alters the membrane conductance in cultured spinal neurons in a fashion similar to flurazepam (MacDonald *et al.*, 1979). On the other hand, benzodiazepine antagonistic properties have also been reported: e.g. inosine antagonizes the anticonvulsive effects of diazepam (Skolnick *et al.*, 1983), antagonizes the effects of diazepam in a behavioural model predictive for anxiolytic activity (Crawley, 1983), and reverses the diazepam-induced decrease of the firing rate of rat substantia nigra zona reticulata neurons (Skolnick *et al.*, 1983). Since the benzodiazepine antagonistic effects are usually seen at much lower inosine concentrations than the agonistic effects, and since inosine binds with considerably higher affinity to the picrotoxin site of the benzodiazepine receptor – GABA receptor – chloride channel complex (Fig. 4.4) than to the benzodiazepine receptor (Olsen, 1982), it has been suggested that the antagonistic effects are mediated via the picrotoxin site and the agonistic effects via the benzodiazepine receptor (Skolnick *et al.*, 1983). However, the affinity of inosine for the benzodiazepine receptor *in vitro* is not affected by GABA and inosine does not enhance GABAergic inhibition *in vivo*, two properties typical for benzodiazepine agonists (Skerritt *et al.*, 1982; Skerritt & MacDonald, 1984). Several other findings also point against a role of inosine as endogenous ligand.

1 The affinity is very low (IC_{50} is about 1 mmol/l) and, together with the low brain levels of about 50 μmol/l (Asano & Spector, 1979; Marangos *et al.*, 1981*b*), a significant *in vivo* occupation of benzodiazepine receptors by this compound appears very unlikely.
2 No evidence exists for the presence of a physiological neuronal

mechanism regulating the brain concentration of inosine (Marangos *et al.*, 1983).

3 The specificity of inosine as a benzodiazepine receptor ligand is quite low and several endogenously occurring purine derivatives inhibit benzodiazepine receptor binding in the same concentration range (Damm *et al.*, 1979; Marangos *et al.*, 1983).

Taking all these findings together, it seems rather unlikely that inosine, or any other purine derivative investigated so far, represents the endogenous ligand of the benzodiazepine receptor. This, however, does not exclude the possibility that purinergic mechanisms regulate benzodiazepine receptor-mediated events as they do in many other neuronal systems of our brain (Snyder, 1985).

Ethyl β-carboline-3-carboxylate

Ethyl β-carboline-3-carboxylate (β-ECC) has been isolated as the active benzodiazepine receptor-binding inhibiting component out of about 1800 litre of human urine (Braestrup *et al.*, 1980; Squires, 1984) and subsequently was identified in rat brain homogenates as well (Braestrup *et al.*, 1980). β-ECC has a very high affinity for the benzodiazepine receptor with an IC_{50} of about 3 nmol/l, similar to many potent benzodiazepine derivatives. It is by far the most potent candidate for the endogenous ligand proposed so far. However, as already mentioned in the first report (Braestrup *et al.*, 1980), β-ECC could not be detected in either human urine or rat brain homogenates unless the isolation procedure included an extraction step using hot, acidic ethanol, a condition which favours the chemical formation of β-ECC from endogenous indole compounds. Accordingly, the present consensus is that β-ECC is a chemical artefact formed from endogenous tryptophan, tryptamine or tryptophan-containing peptides during the isolation procedure (Squires, 1984). It is thus not present in the brain and therefore cannot be considered as an endogenous effector of the benzodiazepine receptor.

On the other hand, the very high affinity of β-ECC and some other β-carboline-3-carboxylates (Braestrup *et al.*, 1980; Lippke *et al.*, 1983) is striking. Moreover, several other β-carboline compounds, including some derivatives physiologically present in mammalian brain, bind with high or intermediate affinity to the benzodiazepine receptor (Rommelspacher *et al.*, 1980, Airaksinen & Kari, 1981; Eder *et al.*, 1981). It is open to question whether the observation about the β-carboline structure fitting so extremely well into the benzodiazepine receptor is mere coincidence or whether this structure represents a link to the putative endogenous effector. This question will be discussed in more detail in a later section of this chapter (§ 6.1.4). Although β-ECC is certainly not the endogenous ligand, its isolation has initiated a vigorous search for structurally related compounds and for their pharmacological properties, which has finally led to the concept of agonists and inverse agonists of the benzodiazepine receptor (see § 4.4). Thus, even if the β-carbolines are not yet linked to an endogenous ligand, the initial findings that β-carbolines bind to the benzodiazepine receptor (Braestrup *et al.*, 1980; Rommelspacher *et al.*, 1980; Airaksinen & Mikkonen, 1980) had a great impact on benzodiazepine receptor research.

Tribulin

Normal human urine contains inhibitory activity for the enzyme monoamine oxidase (MAO). Urinary MAO inhibitory activity is enhanced by stress and physical exercise, shows no selectivity for MAO A or MAO B, and is increased in epileptics and other neurological patients. It has been tentatively termed tribulin (Sandler, 1982, 1983; Sandler *et al.*, 1983; Armando *et al.*, 1984). Tribulin can be extracted into ethyl acetate at pH 1, suggesting acidic or neutral rather than basic properties. However, the chemical nature of tribulin is not yet known, but chromatographic experiments have indicated that it might consist of several low molecular weight fractions (about 300 daltons).

Very interestingly, ethyl acetate extracts of human urine at pH 1 also inhibit benzodiazepine receptor binding *in vitro*, and several experiments indicate that both activities reside in the same material (Sandler, 1983; Sandler *et al.*, 1983; Armando *et al.*, 1984). Accordingly, benzodiazepine receptor-binding inhibiting activity in human urine is increased after stress and physical exercise and is increased in epileptics and other neurological patients with a fairly good linear correlation between both activities (Sandler, 1983). Tribulin is not identical to any other putative candidate for the endogenous ligand tested so far, so its chemical identification remains to be determined.

Referring to recent findings that several inverse agonists of the benzodiazepine receptor with β-carboline structure can induce stress and anxiety in animals and man (File *et al.*, 1982; Dorow *et al.*, 1983) (see also § 6.3), Sandler (1983) has speculated that tribulin might be related to an endogenous anxiety factor acting via the benzodiazepine receptor and bearing structural similarities to β-carbolines. If these speculations can be substantiated experimentally, tribulin could give an important clue to our understanding of physiological mechanisms regulating stress and anxiety in animals and man.

Nephentin

Nephentin, a protein with a molecular weight of about 16 000 daltons, has been found in rat brain extracts and extracts of several other rat tissues (Woolf & Nixon, 1981). It has been isolated and purified to apparent homogeneity from the bile duct of the rat. It has a relatively high affinity for the benzodiazepine receptor, with an IC_{50} of about 50 nmol/l, and does not bind to several other neurotransmitter receptors. Antibodies raised against the purified protein have been used for immunofluorescent experiments indicating a specific staining of neurons located in deep cortical regions of the rat forebrain. While all these findings look quite promising, there is a major drawback in accepting nephentin as endogenous ligand: its tissue distribution in no way mirrors the tissue distribution of benzodiazepine receptors at all. While the benzodiazepine receptor is present only in the CNS, nephentin is present in the rat in nearly all peripheral tissues investigated in even higher concentrations than in the brain, with the highest nephentin level being in the bile duct. Thus, it seems rather unlikely that nephentin itself represents the endogenous ligand. However, it preserves its benzodiazepine receptor-inhibiting properties after extensive proteolytic digestion, suggesting that the major part of the activity can be localized at one or several small proteolytic stable peptides. Accordingly, Woolf & Nixon (1981) have speculated that nephentin might represent a precursor for a lower molecular weight peptide with possible physiological function at the benzodiazepine receptor, but such a nephentin fragment has not yet been isolated.

Other not yet further characterized peptides or proteins

A compound with a molecular weight of about 3000 daltons has been isolated by Davis & Cohen (1980) from bovine brain extracts. It inhibits specific diazepam binding in rat brain membranes competitively, and it has an approximate IC_{50} of around 10 μmol/l. It is relatively heat stable but loses its ability to inhibit benzodiazepine receptor binding after treatment with papain. The peptide nature of the compound was further substantiated by amino acid analysis, indicating the presence of at least eight different amino acids (Davis & Cohen, 1980). Beside its ability to inhibit benzodiazepine receptor binding *in vitro*, the compound also has benzodiazepine-like biological activity in several behavioural tests after intracerebroventricular administration, indicating anticonvulsive and anxiolytic activity (Davis, 1983). Recent data suggest that the 3000 daltons factor is not homogeneous. Thus, the chemical structure of the active fraction (or fractions) and its final status as endogenous ligand remain to be elucidated.

Two fractions which inhibit benzodiazepine receptor binding competitively have been isolated from porcine brain (benzodiazepine-competitive factor, BCF I and II) (Colello *et al.*, 1978). Estimates for their molecular weights range between 1000 and 2000 daltons for BCF II and between 40 000 and 70 000 daltons for BCF I. Neither factor is homogeneous and BCF I contains a major subfraction with a molecular weight of about 60 000 daltons. Both factors are probably proteins, but they have not been further characterized since the first report by Colello

Table 6.4 *Regional distribution of DBI-like immunoreactivity and specific [^{3}H]flunitrazepam binding to benzodiazepine receptors*

Brain region	DBI-like immunoreactivity (pmol/ml protein)*	Specific [^{3}H]FNT binding (fmol/mg protein)†
Arcuate nucleus	350	83
Ventral medial nucleus	190	79
Anterior nucleus	155	68
Medial preoptic area	145	109
Central grey	175	114
Interpeduncular nucleus	170	45
Cerebellar cortex	170	63
Hippocampus, dentate gyros	109	160
Substantia nigra	105	148
Olfactory tubercle	89	31
Globus pallidus	71	70
Nucleus accumbens	60	92
Caudata/putamen	57	76
Frontal cortex	45	213
Occipital cortex	44	131

Note:
*Data from Alho *et al.* (1985).
†Data from Speth *et al.* (1980).

and his colleagues. The status of the factors as endogenous ligands is obscure, especially regarding the unusually large molecular weight of the major component of BCF I. Since serum albumin binds benzodiazepine very strongly (Müller & Wollert, 1973) and also has a molecular weight of about 60 000 daltons, I would like to speculate that the major component of BCF I might be serum albumin, which also interferes with benzodiazepine receptor binding (Braestrup & Squires, 1978).

Another presumably peptide factor with a molecular weight of less than 10 000 daltons has recently been isolated by Wu *et al.* (1984) from rat brain homogenates. Its possible link with one of the other peptides also inhibiting benzodiazepine receptor binding remains to be clarified.

Diazepam displacing activity in human CSF

Kuhn *et al.* (1981) isolated two active fractions from pooled human CSF which inhibited benzodiazepine receptor binding in an agonist-like, GABA-sensitive fashion (see § 4.1.4). The average molecular weights of the two fractions are about 700 or 3600 daltons respectively. No further characteristics of these fractions have yet been reported.

Diazepam binding inhibitor

A polypeptide called diazepam binding inhibitor (DBI) has been isolated and purified to apparent homogeneity from rat brain homogenates (Costa *et al.*, 1983; Guidotti *et al.*, 1983). It has a molecular weight of about 11 000 daltons and inhibits benzodiazepine receptor binding *in vitro* competitively with an IC_{50} of about 4 μmol/l. Its average concentration in rat brain has been estimated as about 10–25 μmol/l (Guidotti *et al.*, 1983). Thus, contrary to most other candidates, this compound has a concentration in the CNS which might be high enough to suggest a relevant benzodiazepine receptor occupation by it *in vivo*. DBI seems to be present only in traces in peripheral organs (liver, kidney, spleen) (Guidotti *et al.*, 1983).

The regional distribution of DBI in the rat CNS has recently been investigated using radioimmuno- and immuno-histochemical methods (Alho *et al.*, 1985). Although DBI-containing neurons might be co-localized with GABAergic neurons in the same brain areas, the regional distribution of DBI-like immunoreactivity does not parallel the regional distribution of the benzodiazepine receptor in the same species (Table 6.4). Although an explanation for this different distribution has not yet been given (Alho *et al.*, 1985), these findings strongly suggest that DBI does not represent the endogenous transmitter ligand of the benzodiazepine receptor, but possibly its precursor.

Similar conclusions have also been drawn on the basis of the relatively large size of DBI and because of its only intermediate affinity for the benzodiazepine receptor. Thus, it has been suggested that the large DBI represents only a precursor molecule of a putative ligand of much smaller molecular weight. In order to identify the sequence of DBI responsible for the interaction with the benzodiazepine receptor, DBI has been fractionated by cyanogen bromide cleavage (Corda *et al.*, 1984) and by tryptic digestion (Ferrero *et al.*, 1984). Benzodiazepine receptor binding activity has been found in fragment F_1 (6500 daltons) containing the amino terminus (cyanogen bromide cleavage) and in a small octadecapeptide found after tryptic digestion. Its sequence is present in fragment F_2 and not in F_1 (cyanogen bromide cleavage). Accordingly, both active peptides are located in different sequences of the precursor DBI. It has been speculated that neither of the two peptides actually represents the endogenous ligand, but that both might contain its final sequence. This would suggest that the putative ligand is a rather small peptide and that DBI acts as precursor for at least two molecules of the final ligand. This might be a frequently observed feature for polypeptides functioning as precursors for peptide transmitters or other neuropeptides (Ferrero *et al.*, 1984).

DBI has been investigated pharmacologically not only with respect to its ability to inhibit benzodiazepine receptor binding but also with respect to its pharmacological profile. The data so far suggest that DBI or its active fragments (see above) are inverse rather than benzodiazepine-like agonists (Costa *et al.*, 1983; Corda *et al.*, 1984; Ferrero *et al.*, 1984). DBI's *in vitro* affinity for the benzodiazepine receptor is not increased by GABA, nor does DBI stimulate GABA receptor binding *in vitro*, two properties typical of benzodiazepine agonists. On the other hand, in the Vogel test (a behavioural paradigm for anxiolytic activity), DBI and its fragments showed proconflict rather than anticonflict properties, similar to the proconflict properties of some inverse agonists with β-carboline structure (Costa *et al.*, 1983). Thus, DBI and its active fragments are anxiogenic rather than anxiolytic, suggesting that the final ligand is an anxiety factor rather than a benzodiazepine-like anti-anxiety or anxiolytic compound. However, these assumptions will remain purely speculative until the final peptide ligand has been unequivocally identified in the brain.

Endogenous benzodiazepine-like immunoreactivity

Benzodiazepine-like immunoreactivity has recently been found in rat brain homogenates by the use of a benzodiazepine-specific monoclonal antibody (Sangameswaran & de Blas, 1985). The tentative molecular weight of the immunoreactive material ranges from 1000 to 300 000 daltons. The antibody used is highly specific for benzodiazepines and does not recognize antagonists like Ro 15–1788 and several β-carbolines. However, its substrate specificity for various benzodiazepines does not correlate with the pharmacological activity (de Blas *et al.*, 1985). These preliminary data again suggest the presence of endogenous compounds with benzodiazepine-like properties of unknown chemical structure. The benzodiazepine-like agonistic properties of this material are also supported by the finding that the binding of these compounds (isolated from rat brain by immunoaffinity chromatography) to the benzodiazepine receptor is enhanced by GABA (Sangameswaran & de Blas, 1985). In conclusion, these data again give some first evidence for the presence of benzodiazepine-like endogenous agonists, suggesting a possible coincidence of these compounds with the 3000 daltons factor (Davis & Cohen, 1980) rather than with DBI (see above).

Summary

Conclusive evidence is present for none of the candidates discussed. For reasons outlined above, the least likely candidates appear to be the small molecular weight compounds nicotinamide, inosine and β-ECC. On the other hand, although DBI obviously does not represent the final active compound, its isolation and that of several similarly active fragments appears to be one of the most promising strategies of the search for the physiological effector molecule. That DBI also represents the precursor for some of the other peptide factors identified so far seems possible, but to what extent has not yet been investigated (e.g. the 3000 dalton factor of Davis & Cohen, 1980). Moreover, if we assume that DBI or its active fragment and the 3000 daltons factor or its active fragment are endogenously present in the brain, we have to assume that the brain contains an anxiety as well as an anti-anxiety factor, both working via the benzodiazepine receptor in a way similar to inverse agonists or agonists respectively. The possible consequences of such an assumption will be discussed at the end of this book (§ 8.2).

6.1.3 *Active compounds present in the brain*

Contrary to the possible candidates described in the preceding part of this chapter, the following substances have not been isolated as active compounds from different biological materials, but have been found by screening many biochemicals normally present in the CNS for biological activity (usually inhibition of benzodiazepine receptor binding). Similar to the candidates described above (§ 6.1.2), their affinities for the benzodiazepine receptor range over at least two orders of magnitude (Table 6.5).

Table 6.5 *Relative receptor affinities of several putative endogenous ligands*

The relative receptor affinities are given as IC_{50} values (inhibitory concentration 50%) and are taken from the references cited in the text. The IC_{50} values of three benzodiazepines are given for comparison. The three drugs approximately represent the affinity range of benzodiazepine drugs acting directly at the receptor.

Compound	IC_{50} (nmol/l)
Nephentin	50
Diazepam binding inhibitor	4 000
Harmane	7 000
Norharmane	8 000
Prostaglandin A_1	7 000
Prostaglandin A_2	15 000
3000 dalton fraction	10 000
L-thyroxine	20 000
Triiodothyronine	33 000
N-acetyl-5-methoxy kynurenamine	65 000
Melatonin	500 000
Inosine	1 300 000
Hypoxanthine	1 300 000
Nicotinamide	4 000 000
Triazolam	1
Diazepam	10
Clobazam	200

Thromboxane A_2

Due to additive effects of two benzodiazepines (diazepam and chlordiazepoxid) and imidazole (a known inhibitor of thromboxane synthetase) on the pressor response to norepinephrine of a rat mesenteric artery preparation, it has been suggested that benzodiazepines might act at a thromboxane A_2 receptor (Ally *et al.*, 1977). There is no further evidence for this, which makes the thromboxane A_2 hypothesis very unlikely.

Prostaglandins

Several prostaglandins (A_1, A_2, B_2) inhibit benzodiazepine receptor binding *in vitro* in the low micromolar range (Asano & Ogasawara, 1982; Matsumoto *et al.*, 1983). Since similar concentrations of these prostaglandins elicit some *in vivo* effects of these compounds, it has been suggested that these substances, which are also present in the CNS, might function endogenously at the benzodiazepine receptor (Asano & Ogasawara, 1982). However, as judged from the GABA shift *in vitro* (see § 4.1.4), the prostaglandins are rather pure benzodiazepine receptor antagonists (Matsumoto *et al.*, 1983), rendering a physiological role very unlikely. Moreover, nothing is known about a functional interaction between prostaglandins and the benzodiazepine receptor–GABA receptor complex, e.g. between prostaglandin synthetase inhibitors like acetylsalicylic acid and benzodiazepines or between benzodiazepine receptor antagonists and prostaglandins in the CNS. Accordingly, the hypothesis that prostaglandins might be the endogenous ligands is also very weak.

Thyroid hormones

L-thyroxine and several other thyroid hormones inhibit benzodiazepine receptor binding *in vitro* with IC_{50} values in the low micromolar range, making these compounds putative candidates for the endogenous ligand (Nagy & Lajtha, 1983). However, endogenous brain levels of the thyroid hormones are much lower than the concentrations needed to inhibit benzodiazepine receptor binding, and the endocrinologically inactive *D*-thyroxine is considerably more active as an inhibitor of benzodiazepine receptor binding than the biologically active *L*-isomer (Nagy & Lajtha,

1983). Thus, little evidence exists at present for relevant physiological effects of thyroid hormones being mediated directly through the benzodiazepine receptor.

Melatonin

Starting with the observation that several β-carbolines bind with intermediate or even high affinity to the benzodiazepine receptor (Airaksinen & Mikkonen, 1980; Braestrup *et al.*, 1980; Rommelspacher *et al.*, 1980), a large variety of other tryptophan-related indole derivatives has been tested for possible affinity for this system (Fehske *et al.*, 1981; Marangos *et al.*, 1981*a*; Lapin, 1983). Out of these compounds, the relatively high affinities of melatonin and especially of its brain metabolite *N*-acetyl-5-methoxy-kynurenamine are striking. Again, however, the IC_{50}s are not high enough to suggest a physiological relevance of these observations, especially if one looks for the brain concentrations of the two compounds.

Harmane and norharmane

Several years ago we observed a stereoselective competition between benzodiazepines and *L*-tryptophan for the indole binding site of human serum albumin (Müller & Wollert, 1973, 1975, 1979), suggesting structural similarities between benzodiazepines and tryptophan analogues. Accordingly, a large variety of tryptophan and indole derivatives was tested for possible binding to the benzodiazepine receptor. While most of these compounds turned out to have only a low affinity for this system (Fehske *et al.*, 1981), a few β-carboline derivatives, especially harmane and norharmane, showed relatively high affinities (Rommelspacher *et al.*, 1980). Similar observations were made independently by Airaksinen & Mikkonen (1980). Subsequent studies indicated that both compounds also interact with the benzodiazepine receptor *in vivo* after i.v. or i.p. administration to rats or mice (Morin *et al.*, 1981; Fehske & Müller, 1982). In pharmacological tests, harmane showed convulsive (Rommelspacher *et al.*, 1981) and anxiogenic (Rommelspacher *et al.*, 1982) properties, which can be antagonized by low doses of benzodiazepines. A slightly different profile has been found for norharmane (Morin *et al.*, 1981; Rommelspacher *et al.*, 1981). In addition, norharmane has been demonstrated to produce kindling of seizures when given chronically (Morin *et al.*, 1983; Morin, 1984). The mechanism is very likely to be mediated through the benzodiazepine receptor, since kindling by norharmane can be prevented not only by benzodiazepines but also by the benzodiazepine receptor antagonist Ro 15–1788. Thus, both β-carbolines have pharmacological properties indicative of inverse rather than benzodiazepine-like agonistic properties (see § 4.4). However, since both compounds lack a high degree of specificity for the benzodiazepine receptor, the participation of other neuronal systems in their mechanism of action cannot be excluded (Müller *et al.*, 1981).

In the light of previous findings about the presence of harmane in rat brain and in human urine and blood (Rommelspacher *et al.*, 1980, 1984), this compound should be considered as a putative candidate for the endogenous ligand. Its regional distribution in the rat brain parallels the regional distribution of the benzodiazepine receptor to some extent, with high levels in the cortex, cerebellum and hippocampus, and much lower levels in the striatum and the hypothalamus (Rommelspacher *et al.*, 1984). Its basal level in many areas of the rat brain, however, is about 20 nmol/l (Rommelspacher *et al.*, 1984). Considering its *in vitro* affinity for the benzodiazepine receptor of about 7 μmol/l (Rommelspacher *et al.*, 1980), the brain concentration is probably too low to suggest the possibility of a physiologically relevant benzodiazepine receptor occupation *in vivo* by harmane. These findings and the complete lack of data about possible storage or release mechanisms of harmane in the brain strongly point against harmane as the endogenous ligand. On the other hand, harmane is present in the brain and it has at least some pharmacological properties mediated through the benzodiazepine receptor. Thus, harmane might be an important link in suggesting a possible relevance of the β-carboline nucleus as part of the chemical structure of the putative ligand.

Summing up

None of these candidates represents the endogenous ligand. If there is any possible clue to an endogenous ligand, it is again the connection to the β-carboline structure.

6.1.4 *The biomimetic approach*

As already mentioned, several β-carbolines seem to fit very well into the benzodiazepine receptor, but none of them represents the endogenous ligand because of their low concentration or even absence in the brain. Moreover, for β-ECC or related compounds, even the presence of a biosynthetic pathway seems to be very unlikely. On the other hand, by assuming the β-carboline structure as a biologically feasible model compound, several β-carboline-related structures have been synthesized and investigated as possible ligands of the benzodiazepine receptor. Since, for all these compounds, a biosynthetic pathway might be present in the CNS, this approach has been termed 'biomimetic' by Guzman *et al.* (1984).

Although not all steps of the biosynthesis of harmane and norharmane are yet finally known, it is generally assumed that these compounds are biochemically formed by a Pictet–Spengler condensation of indoleamines or tryptophan with aldehydes, usually formaldehyde in the case of norharmane and acetaldehyde in the case of harmane (Airaksinen & Kari, 1981; Rommelspacher, 1981). It has been suggested that similar condensation products might also occur with higher aldehydes, originated from the Krebs cycle (Guzman *et al.*, 1984). One of these compounds, a condensation product originating from tryptamine and γ-ketoglutaric acid (a canthin-6-one derivative), shows relatively high affinity for the benzodiazepine receptor with an IC_{50} of about 100 nmol/l (Guzman *et al.*, 1984). Although such derivatives occur only in plants and not in mammalian bodies, this approach could give some hints for putative endogenously occurring compounds with high affinities for the benzodiazepine receptor.

Our own studies using this approach are directed at the search for β-carboline derivatives which, in contrast to the β-carboline-3-carboxylates (Lippke *et al.*, 1983), not only exhibit a high affinity for the benzodiazepine receptor, but also possess chemical structures which can be formed by biochemical pathways. A few years ago we found relatively low affinities for several tryptophan-containing dipeptides (Fehske *et al.*, 1981), but considerably higher affinities were reported by Eder *et al.* (1981) for some β-carboline-3-carboxamides, including the glycine derivative. Contrary to the β-carboline-3-carboxylates, a biochemical pathway is feasible for β-carboline-3-carboxamides if physiological amino acids are assumed to be the amine component. It also seems possible that the β-carboline structure is formed *in vivo* from *N*-terminal tryptophan residues of small peptides. In any case, the resulting compounds will represent small peptides, blocked at the *N*-terminal site by a β-carboline residue. While our data obtained so far (Lippke *et al.*, 1985, 1987) do not yet indicate derivatives with very high affinities, many β-carboline-3-carboxamides from *L*-amino acids as the amine component bind to the benzodiazepine receptor with affinities in the range of that of harmane itself (Lippke *et al.*, 1985). Moreover, the affinity can be increased by increasing the molecular size, e.g. by changing from di- to tri- or tetra-peptides (Lippke *et al.*, 1987). It seems that these larger molecules are able to bind to a further point of attachment, presumably located outside the recognition site of the benzodiazepine receptor for the β-carboline nucleus (Lippke *et al.*, 1985).

In conclusion, although the biomimetic approach has also not yet given a final structure, it suggests the possibility of an endogenous ligand representing a small peptide, blocked at the *N*-terminus by a β-carboline structure, presumably formed from an *N*-terminal tryptophan residue.

6.1.5 *Many interesting compounds, but not yet an endogenous ligand*

As outlined above, the search for an endogenous benzodiazepine has produced a large variety of interesting compounds, but not yet the putative ligand. If one attempts to make some kind of synopsis, two observations are particularly striking. Of all the compounds isolated from biological materials, DBI fulfils most but certainly not all of the criteria of an endogenously relevant compound, possibly functioning as a precursor molecule. At least one of its possible active fragments has its *N*-terminus blocked. On the other hand, the relatively high affinity of some β-carbolines, as members of a biologically occurring class of compounds, is quite remarkable. Moreover, our own data suggest that the β-carboline structure can be incorporated as the *N*-terminal part in small di-, tri- or tetra-peptides without reducing and even slightly increasing the benzodiazepine receptor affinity. Thus, one feels entitled to speculate that the *N*-terminal block of the DBI molecule could represent a similarly positioned β-carboline nucleus.

Interestingly, the highest concentrations of DBI (Alho *et al.*, 1985) as well as of harmane (Shoemaker *et al.*, 1980), one of the few β-carbolines present in the mammalian brain (Airaksinen & Kari, 1981), have been found for the rat CNS in the arcuate nucleus of the hypothalamus. Moreover, the regional distribution of harmane in the rat brain (Rommelspacher *et al.*, 1984) shows some similarities to that of DBI (Alho *et al.*, 1985), except in the cortex, where high harmane but low DBI levels have been found. Thus, brain areas where DBI is present might be able to synthesize β-carbolines. Accordingly, it might be worth while to investigate further the possible relevance of the β-carboline structure as part of a peptide ligand of the benzodiazepine receptor.

On the other hand, beside this speculation, our general failure to identify the putative ligand could alternatively be interpreted as evidence that such an endogenous benzodiazepine does not exist. Since evidence for the presence of an endogenously acting compound can also be obtained indirectly, e.g. from experiments with antagonists, the next parts of this chapter review our present knowledge about the important question of whether we have to assume the presence of an endogenous effector at the benzodiazepine receptor from studies with pure antagonists.

6.2 Effects of benzodiazepine receptor antagonists on neuronal activity, sleep, and behaviour indicative of the presence of an endogenous ligand

The development of benzodiazepine receptor antagonists (see § 3.4) has given the experimental basis for this pharmacological approach, assuming that when administered alone, such antagonists should also antagonize the effects of a putative physiological receptor ligand. Accordingly, the pharmacological properties of such an antagonist should be explainable by an inhibition of the effects of the endogenous effector, as is the case for atropine at the muscarin cholinergic receptor. This approach has one major handicap: if one assumes that the physiological role of the natural benzodiazepine receptor ligand is present only under certain specific conditions and even then is not of primary relevance for CNS function, only small pharmacological effects can be observed after the administration of such an antagonist. Hence, it can be very difficult to decide if the effects observed can be explained by an antagonism of an endogenous effector or by traces of agonistic (intrinsic) activity of the antagonist used (as is the case for Ro 15–1788). Both problems can be clearly demonstrated using the example of opiate antagonists and their effects on the endogenous opiate system.

Pure opiate antagonists like naloxone have been considered for many years as being devoid of intrinsic pharmacological properties, thus giving no evidence for the presence of endogenous opiates. However, starting with the discovery of the opiate receptor and the subsequent identification of endogenous opiate-like compounds (endorphins) and their physiological role in regulating pain, the pharmacological properties of naloxone have been reinvestigated in animals and man under experimental conditions thought to activate the endorphin-containing neuronal system regulating pain sensations (Watkins & Mayer, 1982). And, indeed, under certain specific noxious stimuli, a small but distinct hyperalgesic effect of naloxone could be demonstrated in experimental animals and man (Fields & Levine, 1984). This suggests that the endogenous endorphinergic system is activated only under very specific conditions. Even then, its physiological function (analgesia) is not very pronounced and its quantification requires very specific experimental settings (Watkins & Mayer, 1982; Fields & Levine, 1984). If these findings are transferred to the field of benzodiazepine receptor research, they might suggest that the lack of pharmacological properties of benzodiazepine receptor antagonists under normal experimental conditions is not necessarily indicative of the absence of physiological ligands.

Indeed, most previous investigations about the pharmacology of the rather 'pure' antagonist Ro 15–1788 indicated the absence of intrinsic activity in animals and man at doses high enough to occupy a significant percentage of benzodiazepine receptors *in vivo* (Hunkeler *et al.*, 1981; Polc *et al.*, 1981; Darragh *et al.*, 1983). All these experiments have been performed under normal experimental settings and suggest that, even if present, a putative endogenous ligand of the benzodiazepine receptor is not of major relevance for CNS function. However, as already outlined for the effects of naloxone on the endogenous pain sensations regulating system, it can be speculated that a putative endogenous 'benzodiazepinergic' system is also only activated after certain specific stimuli. Accordingly, if one looks very carefully over the literature on this aspect, some evidence emerges for the presence of endogenous benzodiazepine receptor ligands. Again, the question of possible intrinsic activities of the antagonists employed is of major importance. Therefore, for most studies the Roche compound Ro 15–1788 has been used, since its properties come closest to those of a 'pure' antagonist, although some agonistic (benzodiazepine-like) properties are present. These, however, are seen only when high doses are used.

6.2.1 *Effects on neuronal activity*

Initial electrophysiological studies showed no effects of Ro 15–1788 on the excitability of central neurons (Polc *et al.*, 1981), but some subsequent investigations indicated that this compound can affect central excitability in a benzodiazepine-opposite way by decreasing GABAergic inhibition (Carlen *et al.*, 1983; Krespan *et al.*, 1984). It is interesting that these effects are much more pronounced for physiologically released GABA than for exogenously applied GABA (Krespan *et al.*, 1984). This observation has been interpreted as indicating the presence of a benzodiazepine-like endogenous compound which is co-released after various stimuli and facilitates GABAergic inhibition (Krespan *et al.*, 1984). Its antagonism by Ro 15–1788 decreases GABAergic inhibition. This effect, however, was only slight and could not be observed for every hippocampal slice preparation investigated. Accordingly, the authors stated 'if endogenous benzodiazepine-agonist ligands are present, they play at most a small role in modulating the actions of GABA in the hypothalamus or hippocampus following electrical stimulation' (Krespan *et al.*, 1984).

6.2.2 *Studies on animal behaviour*

As in the electrophysiological studies, initial studies with Ro 15–1788 showed little if any intrinsic behavioural effects (Boast *et al.*, 1983; Haefely, 1983). Also similar to the electrophysiological studies, subsequent experiments, using more sophisticated experimental designs, revealed slight agonistic properties in most behavioural paradigms (at least at high doses), but also some inverse agonistic properties in some other paradigms (mostly at lower doses). Since a slight benzodiazepine-like intrinsic activity of Ro 15–1788 is known, the agonistic effects of Ro 15–1788 on animal behaviour are easily explained on this basis (Haefely, 1983; Jensen *et al.*, 1984). This property of Ro 15–1788 does not explain the inverse agonistic effects (proconvulsive, anxiogenic), which have been seen mainly for low doses of this drug. These observations, however, can be very easily explained if one assumes the presence of an endogenous benzodiazepine, which is antagonized by Ro 15–1788 (Pellow, 1985). Again, its modulating function on GABAergic inhibition seems to be only of secondary relevance, so that the inhibition of this system by Ro 15–1788 results in only minor but distinct disturbances of CNS function. On the other hand, if GABAergic neurotransmission is partially impaired by isoniazide, which depletes neuronal storage mechanisms of GABA in the CNS, the proconvulsive and anxiogenic properties of Ro 15–1788 are much more pronounced (Corda *et al.*, 1982; Lal & Harris, 1985). Thus, when GABAergic inhibition is pathologically decreased, the regulating function of the putative endogenous benzodiazepine receptor ligand might become functionally more relevant.

Evidence for the presence of a benzodiazepine-like endogenous ligand has also been presented very recently in a study on the effects of ZK 93 426, a β-carboline benzodiazepine receptor antagonist (Jensen *et al.*, 1984), in two animal tests predictive of anxiety (File *et al.*, 1986).

Taking all the present evidence together, the reported effects of benzodiazepine receptor antagonists on animal behaviour support rather than disprove the presence of an endogenous benzodiazepine receptor ligand, as has been summarized recently by File & Pellow (1986).

6.2.3 *Effects on behaviour and sleep in humans*

Initial studies with the rather 'pure' benzodiazepine receptor antagonist Ro 15–1788 in humans did not indicate any intrinsic activity of this drug with respect to cognitive, psychomotor and subjective functions or in relation to the electroencephalographic pattern (Darragh *et al.*, 1983; Gath *et al.*, 1984). Similar to the experiments in animals, subsequent studies using more sophisticated experimental designs did, however, reveal some intrinsic effects of this compound in man.

Schöpf *et al* (1984) investigated the effects of a single intravenous dose of 5 mg Ro 15–1788 on the electroencephalogram of 10 healthy volunteers. The effects seen on the EEG are consistent with the assumption that this drug has a central activating effect, similar but not identical to that of some nootropics or psychostimulants. Similarly, in our recent study about the effects of an oral dose of 30 mg of Ro 15–1788 on healthy volunteers, evidence for a centrally activating but rather dysphoric effect has been found using several psychometric tests (Zimmer *et al.*, 1986). On the other hand, after a night of sleep withdrawal, no effect of 10 mg of Ro 15–1788 administered intravenously was observed in a study on five healthy volunteers using several psychometric tests. In three of the five subjects, however, an increase of anxiety was found by a self-rating test (Emrich *et al.*, 1984).

Evidence for a central activating effect of Ro 15–1788 in man also comes from sleep studies. Gaillard & Blois (1983) found only a slight effect of an evening dose of 100 mg Ro 15–1788 (orally) on sleep parameters of 12 healthy volunteers. There was a tendency for a reduction of many sleep parameters, but the only significant change was a reduction of the mean duration of the sleep cycles. Similarly, no significant effects on human sleep parameters have been found in a recent study on the effects of 40 mg Ro 15–1788 given orally at bedtime to five volunteers after one night of sleep withdrawal (Emrich & Lund, 1985). Since the elimination half-life of Ro 15–1788 in man is less than 1 h (Klotz *et al.*, 1984), few effects of this drug on whole night sleep parameters can be expected when this drug is given once at bedtime. This handicap of the two latter studies is not present in a recent study by Ziegler *et al.* (1985), where 10 mg Ro 15–1788 was administered intravenously to volunteers at sleep during the first time they reached stage 3. The sleep parameters were monitored not only for the whole night but also for the first hour after the administration of the drug or placebo. Similar to the two other investigations, few effects were seen on whole night sleep parameters, although a tendency for a reduction of stage 4 sleep was present. By contrast, if sleep parameters were calculated for the first hour after administration only, Ro 15–1788 was highly effective when compared with placebo (double-blind design) and decreased nearly all sleep parameters significantly, indicating benzodiazepine-opposite, centrally activating properties (Ziegler *et al.*, 1985). A comparable observation has been reported by Wauquier & Ashton (1984) in dogs, where Ro 15–1788 changed the sleep EEG in a way opposite to that of benzodiazepines.

Again, the effects of Ro 15–1788 are compatible with the assumption of an antagonism of an endogenous benzodiazepine by this drug and with the assumption that this putative endogenous benzodiazepine plays only a secondary role for central function in man as in animals.

6.2.4 *Effects on hepatic coma in man*

One of the first clinical studies with Ro 15–1788 indicated its rapid effectiveness in reversing coma due to benzodiazepine overdosage (Scollo-Lavizzari, 1983). In subsequent studies, two groups also reported a stimulant effect of Ro 15–1788 in coma due to hepatic encephalopathy in patients who had obviously been free of any benzodiazepine medication for several days (Bansky *et al.*, 1985; Scollo-Lavizzari & Steinmann, 1985). Injections of very low doses of Ro 15–1788 (between 0.3 and 0.5 mg) to deep comatose (stage 3 but mainly stage 4) patients resulted in remarkable improvements. The patients became responsive again with a parallel improvement of the pathological EEG. The improvement usually lasted about 1 h in all patients, after which time the patients became comatose again. In some patients, the effect of Ro 15–1788 could be reproduced by repeated injections of the same drug but not by injections of naloxone or physostigmine. These findings strongly suggest that the stimulant effect of Ro 15–1788 in the comatose patients is related to its benzodiazepine receptor blocking properties. Since the patients have been free of any benzodiazepine medication for several days, it seems rather unlikely that these observations can be explained by an antagonism of benzodiazepines present in the CNS, although the impaired elimination of some benzodiazepines during hepatic dysfunction has to be considered.

These findings strongly suggest antagonism of an endogenous benzodiazepine-like compound by low doses of Ro 15–1788. The much higher activity of Ro 15–1788 in comatose patients than in healthy volunteers could indicate either an elevated CNS concentration of the putative ligand or an increased sensitivity of the benzodiazepine receptor. Very interestingly, supersensitivity of the benzodiazepine receptor has been reported for an animal model of hepatic encephalopathy in rabbits and rats (Schafer *et al.*, 1983; Baraldi *et al.*, 1984). Moreover, pronounced disturbances of GABAergic transmission have also been found in the same animal models of hepatic encephalopathy (Baraldi & Zeneroli, 1982). Both observations could support the hypothesis that the putative endogenous benzodiazepine is functionally much more relevant in situations where GABAergic transmission is disturbed. Furthermore, it is an old clinical observation that patients with liver disease are much more sensitive to benzodiazepines than subjects with normal liver function, an observation obviously due not only to the reduced hepatic elimination of the drugs, but also to an increased sensitivity of the brain for the benzodiazepines (Fisch *et al.*, 1986). These observations also suggest an increased sensitivity of the benzodiazepine receptor system in hepatic diseases.

To what extent the recently reported beneficial effect of the benzodiazepine receptor antagonist Ro 15–1788 in cases of isolated ethanol intoxications can also be explained by sensitivity changes of the benzodiazepine receptor or by altered levels of a putative endogenous ligand is at present not known (Scollo-Lavizzari & Matthis, 1985).

6.2.5 *Effects on seizure activity in epileptic patients*

In a preliminary report, Scollo-Lavizzari (1984) found an anticonvulsive effect of relatively low doses of Ro 15–1788 in a small number of epileptic patients who were obviously free of any medication with benzodiazepines. This finding parallels some other findings about the anticonvulsive activity of low doses of Ro 15–1788 in various animal tests for seizure activity (File & Pellow, 1986). Because of the low doses used, it seems unlikely that these observations can be explained by the small intrinsic benzodiazepine-like agonistic properties of this compound, which are usually thought to explain anticonvulsive properties of Ro 15–1788 given at very high doses (File & Pellow, 1986). Thus, the small anticonvulsive effects of low doses of Ro 15–1788 in animals and man might indicate the presence of an endogenous inverse agonist of the benzodiazepine receptor, whose convulsive or proconvulsive properties are antagonized by the benzodiazepine receptor antagonist Ro 15–1788. It is important to note that this assumption is different from most other findings using Ro 15–1788 at low doses, which usually indicate the presence of an endogenous compound with benzodiazepine-like properties.

6.2.6 *Do we have conclusive proof for the presence of an endogenous benzodiazepine from studies with antagonists?*

As outlined above, many recent studies using the relatively 'pure' benzodiazepine receptor antagonist Ro 15–1788 are consistent with the assumption of the presence of an endogenous benzodiazepine-like compound in the brains of animals and man. Its physiological function, however – and that seems to be a very important point – is at most only of secondary relevance for our CNS, but might become more important in certain situations, e.g. when GABAergic transmission is generally impaired.

There is one alternative explanation for the slight CNS-stimulating properties of Ro 15–1788, assuming that this drug behaves at low doses like an inverse benzodiazepine receptor antagonist and only at high doses as a benzodiazepine-like agonist. In addition to the fact that such pharmacological properties would require a very complicated mechanism of action at the receptor level, this putative explanation could not account for the findings that the slight CNS-stimulating properties of Ro 15–1788 are more pronounced for endogenously present than for exogenously applied GABA. Thus, the first assumption represents the much more simple mechanism and fits nicely into the hypothesis of an endogenous effector as a co-transmitter for GABAergic transmission (see § 8.2).

6.3 Does one of the pharmacological properties of benzodiazepine receptor agonists or inverse agonists mirror a specific CNS function in animals or man?

One of the important and fundamental criteria to identify the possible neurotransmitter function of a given substance is the requirement that its effects on a specific organ or on a specific neuron should mimic physiological activity. Accordingly, if we ask for the possible endogenous function of the benzodiazepine receptor, one important criterion could be that its stimulation by agonists (or inverse agonists) mimics a certain aspect of physiological brain function or even dysfunction. The latter case is explained best using as an example the observations that chronic treatment with amphetamine (and to a much smaller extent with *L*-dopa) can result in schizophreniform psychoses, one of the major arguments for the dopamine hypothesis of at least type I schizophrenia (Crow, 1982).

Up to now, there is little evidence that one of the classical pharmacological properties of the benzodiazepines mimics the stimulation of the benzodiazepine receptor by an endogenous compound. Thus, these effects might represent unspecific stimulation of benzodiazepine receptors in many brain regions, rather than the activation of only a certain number of receptors involved in the regulation of a specific aspect of brain function. Similarly, many of the pharmacological properties of inverse agonists of the benzodiazepine receptor suggest unspecific CNS stimulation rather than the activation of a specific neuronal system of the CNS (Haefely, 1983; Nutt, 1983).

One possible exception might be the β-carboline model of anxiety (Insel *et al.*, 1984; Skolnick *et al.*, 1984), indicating the specific involvement of benzodiazepine receptor ligands in the regulation of fear and anxiety. Making the assumption that inverse agonists should have pharmacological properties opposite to those of the classical agonists (benzodiazepines), e.g. anxiogenic versus anxiolytic, Skolnick *et al.* (1984) used β-ECC (a weak inverse agonist of the benzodiazepine receptor) for a chemically induced animal model of human anxiety. Within minutes after the intravenous injection of β-ECC to rhesus monkeys, a behavioural syndrome very much reminiscent of fear and anxiety was observed (Table 6.6), which was not found for animals receiving the vehicle only. Moreover, these behavioural changes were accompanied by a variety of somatic symptoms typical for intense anxiety states in animals or man, including increased heart rate and blood pressure and elevated plasma concentrations of adrenocorticotrophic hormone (ACTH), cortisol, epinephrine, and norepinephrine (Skolnick *et al.*, 1984). Behavioural and somatic symptoms could be specifically blocked by diazepam as well as by the pure

Table 6.6 *The behavioural effects of* β-*ECC (2.5 mg/kg i.v.) within 2 h after infusion in the rhesus monkey*

Behaviour	Vehicle ($n = 7$)	β-ECC ($n = 7$)
Agitation (struggling in chair)	0	7
Increased head and body turning	0	7
Immobility (5 s)	1	7
Bleeding caused by scratching	0	2
Eating and drinking	7	0
Distress vocalization	0	6
Defaecation and urination immediately after infusion	0	7
Penile erection immediately after infusion	0	7
Sedation	1	2

Source: Data are taken from Skolnick *et al.* (1984).

benzodiazepine receptor antagonist Ro 15–1788. Thus, the data strongly suggest that the interaction of the inverse agonist β-ECC with the benzodiazepine receptor produces a variety of behavioural and somatic symptoms typical for intense levels of anxiety and fear. However, the problem with this model is that the monkeys obviously cannot say whether the feeling of fear and anxiety in these chemically induced behavioural states is similar to the feeling of physiological situations of fear or anxiety.

On the other hand, the β-ECC-induced model of anxiety gains some support from preliminary data about a β-carboline-induced anxiety syndrome in man (Dorow *et al.*, 1983). The authors reported very similar symptoms in two healthy volunteers after the injection of the chemically closely related compound, β-carboline monomethylamide (FG 7142), including intense feelings of anxiety and fear accompanied by the increases of blood pressure, heart rate and plasma cortisol. These symptoms could be blocked immediately by the intravenous administration of a benzodiazepine.

While these data in animals and man suggest strongly that the activation of benzodiazepine receptors with inverse agonists induces a pattern of behavioural and somatic symptoms closely resembling those of physiological fear and anxiety, there is little evidence that a similar mechanism is generally involved in these emotions. Most arguments for the latter assumption come from studies with the pure antagonist Ro 15–1788, which shows an anxiogenic effect rather than an anxiolytic effect in some animal models of anxiety (Pellow, 1985). This is the opposite of the effect one would predict if the activation of benzodiazepine receptors by an (endogenous) inverse agonist is of major importance for mediating physiological fear and anxiety. Thus, the β-carboline-induced model of anxiety could alternatively be explained by an unspecific CNS stimulation by this inverse agonist, since anxiogenic effects have also been reported for a variety of CNS stimulants or convulsives when used at relatively low doses (Pellow, 1985). On the other hand, additional evidence for the involvement of an endogenous inverse agonist of the benzodiazepine receptor in the neuronal mechanisms leading to anxiety and fear comes from the experiments on stress and electrical foot-shocks on low-affinity GABA receptors, effects which can be mimicked by β-carbolines and which can be blocked by the pure benzodiazepine receptor antagonist Ro 15–1788 (see § 7.2.3). It is also supported by very recent data showing that a benzodiazepine receptor mechanism is involved in the stress-induced secretion of β-endorphin from the rat pituitary (Maiewski *et al.*, 1985).

Thus, while some data suggest that benzodiazepine receptor mechanisms are in some way involved in the physiological regulation of fear and anxiety in animals and man, these effects are certainly not the major endogenous mechanisms of the two emotions.

6.4 Benzodiazepine receptor up- and down-regulation: an indication for receptor super- or sub-sensitivity?

Increasing evidence has accumulated over the last decade that alterations of neurotransmitter receptors are involved in the phenomenon of denervation supersensitivity as well as in the phenomenon of subsensitivity after a prolonged period of neuronal activity. Usually, conditions which chronically decrease the interaction of a given neurotransmitter with its synaptic receptor will increase the sensitivity of the postsynaptic cell (supersensitivity). One of the mechanisms possible is an increase of the number of postsynaptic receptors. Conversely, conditions which chronically increase the interaction of a given neurotransmitter with its receptor decrease the sensitivity of the postsynaptic cell (subsensitivity). Again, one of the mechanisms possible is a decrease of the number of postsynaptic receptors. The two phenomena, also called up- and down-regulation respectively, develop very slowly (within days) after changing the synaptic activity and might be due to changes of protein synthesis or degradation, or develop very rapidly (within minutes) and may possibly be explained by receptor internalization. The functional significance of such alterations of the number of receptors, usually determined by direct binding experiments, for the activity of synaptic transmission is not always clear, since such alterations are only part of the adaptive changes regulating over- or under-activity of neuronal functions. The specific aspects of receptors' up- or down-regulation as parts of the phenomena of super- or sub-sensitivity of chemical neurotransmission have been reviewed by Overstreet & Yamamura (1979), Enna (1984), and Schweitzer *et al.* (1984). Today, there is no doubt that such changes of neuroreceptors represent an integral part of the physiological mechanisms regulating synaptic transmission. Thus, if similar regulative changes of the benzodiazepine receptor in terms of super- or sub-sensitivity could be demonstrated conclusively, the possible physiological function of this system would be strongly supported. Such data, however, should be reviewed very carefully, as they might simply mirror adaptive changes of the whole benzodiazepine receptor–GABA receptor complex, thus representing super- or sub-sensitivity of GABAergic transmission rather than of the benzodiazepine receptor. Accordingly, special attention will be paid to those adaptive changes where the GABA receptor and the benzodiazepine receptor are regulated independently.

6.4.1 *Chronic treatment with agonists (benzodiazepines)*

Chronic treatment with usually very high daily doses of several benzodiazepines results in a down-regulation of benzodiazepine receptor density in rats and mice in agreement with the notion of benzodiazepines acting as agonists (Table 6.7). The effect is more pronounced in the frontal

Table 6.7 *Benzodiazepine receptor up- and down-regulation by chronic treatment with agonists or antagonists*

Animals were treated for the time indicated with the drugs. Benzodiazepine receptor properties were determined by Scatchard analyses. Changes in receptor density are given as percentage changes of B_{max}. Relevant changes of the receptor affinity were usually not found.

Days of treatment	Daily dose (mg/kg)	Species	Brain region	% change of B_{max}	Reference
28	Diazepam (4)	Rat	Several	±0	Möhler *et al.* (1978)
56	Diazepam (90) Lorazepam (60)	Rat Rat	Forebrain Cortex	±0 −18	Braestrup *et al.* (1978)
10	Flurazepam (100)	Rat	Cortex	−15	Chiu & Rosenberg (1978)
28	Flurazepam (150)	Rat	Cortex Hippocampus Striatum Cerebellum	−14 −17 ±0 ±0	Rosenberg & Chiu (1981)
14	Diazepam (5)	Rat	Cortex	−14	Grimm & Hershkowitz (1981)
20	Clonazepam (15)	Mouse	Forebrain	−46	Crawley *et al.* (1982)
14	Diazepam (4)	Rat	Cortex	±0	Medina *et al.* (1983*b*)
8	β-ECC, intraventricularly	Rat	Cortex Cerebellum Hippocampus	+63 +51 +38	Concas *et al.* (1983)
14	Ro 15–1788 (4)	Rat	Cortex Hippocampus	+26 +23	Medina *et al.* (1983*a*)

cortex and the hippocampus than in the cerebellum and the striatum and is not seen for chronic treatment with low doses of benzodiazepines, e.g. 4 mg/kg diazepam daily (Table 6.7). The down-regulation of benzodiazepine receptor density does not persist for a long time after cessation of chronic treatment, and benzodiazepine receptor levels are usually normal again after only a few days (Rosenberg & Chiu, 1981; Crawley *et al.*, 1982). This explains the negative findings of Braestrup *et al.* (1978), although very high doses of benzodiazepines were used (Table 6.7), since the binding studies were performed 11 days after the last treatment. Using similar experimental settings, the authors found a decrease of the density by about 21% for both treatments, when binding was assayed 5 days after the last administration of the drugs (Braestrup *et al.*, 1978).

A similar down-regulation has been found in most studies using cell cultures of fetal mouse brain or spinal cord chronically exposed to diazepam (Table 6.8). As in the *in vivo* experiments, the diazepam concentration was usually quite high and above therapeutically relevant concentrations. One exception is the recent report by Sher (1983), who found a benzodiazepine receptor down-regulation of about 70% in tissue cultures of fetal mouse cerebral cortex exposed for 10 days to a diazepam concentration of about 450 ng/ml, which is within the therapeutically relevant range. This appears to be the only study indicating benzodiazepine

Table 6.8 *Effect of chronic exposure to benzodiazepines on benzodiazepine receptor binding to tissue cultures*

Tissue cultures were exposed for the time indicated to diazepam in the concentration given. Benzodiazepine receptor properties were determined by Scatchard analyses. Changes in receptor density are given as percentage changes of B_{max}. Relevant changes of the receptor affinity have not been found.

Days of exposure	Drug concentration	Tissue culture	% change of B_{max}	Reference
21	Diazepam (1 μmol/l)	Fetal mouse brain	± 0	Shibla *et al.* (1981)
5	Diazepam (10 μmol/l)	Fetal mouse brain	–20	Prezioso & Neale (1983)
7	Diazepam (13 μmol/l)	Fetal mouse spinal cord	–20	Sher *et al.* (1983)
10	Diazepam (1.5 μmol/l)	Fetal mouse cortex	–70	Sher (1983)
10	Diazepam (6.3 μmol/l)	Fetal mouse cortex	–99	Sher (1983)

receptor down-regulation by therapeutic concentrations of a benzodiazepine.

While the data reported in Table 6.7 agree with the assumption of benzodiazepine receptor subsensitivity as often observed after chronic overstimulation of a given neurotransmitter system, they could indicate alternatively subsensitivity of the GABAergic system mediated by down-regulation of the whole benzodiazepine receptor–GABA receptor complex. Experimental evidence, however, speaks clearly against this assumption (Table 6.9), indicating that the properties of the GABA receptor change in a fashion opposite to that of the benzodiazepine receptor after chronic benzodiazepine treatment. Although it is not possible at present to explain these findings in terms of synaptic function, they strongly suggest that benzodiazepine receptor subsensitivity is a specific response to chronic treatment with benzodiazepines and is not parallelled by similar changes of the GABA receptor. In this respect, it is important to note that not only

Table 6.9 *GABA receptor up-regulation by chronic treatment with benzodiazepines*

Animals were treated with the drugs for the time indicated. GABA receptor properties were determined from Scatchard analyses. Changes in receptor density are given as percentage changes of B_{max}.

Days of treatment	Daily dose (mg/kg)	Species	Brain region	% change of B_{max}	Reference
20	Clonazepam (15)	Mouse	Forebrain Cerebellum	+19[a] +27	Marangos & Crawley (1982)
20	Chlordiazepoxid (15)	Mouse	Forebrain Cerebellum	+ 6[a] +27	Marangos & Crawley (1982)
21	Chlordiazepoxid (0.22)	Rat	Cortex	+180[b] + 15[c]	Abbracchio *et al.* (1983)
21	Chlordiazepoxid (2.6)	Rat	Cortex	+390[d] +680[e]	Abbracchio *et al.* (1983)

Note:
[a]High-affinity [^{3}H]muscimol binding, K_D remains unchanged. Under the same conditions, B_{max} of specific [^{3}H]flunitrazepam binding was reduced by about 40%.
[b,c]Represent high- and low-affinity components of [^{3}H]GABA binding respectively, K_D was also increased four- and six-fold respectively. Under the same conditions, B_{max} of specific [^{3}H]flunitrazepam binding was reduced by about 60%.
[d,e]Represent high- and low-affinity components of [^{3}H]GABA binding respectively, K_D was also increased ten- and six-fold respectively. Under the same conditions, B_{max} of specific [^{3}H]flunitrazepam binding was reduced by about 40%.

the high-affinity but also the low-affinity GABA receptors are up-regulated after chronic treatment with benzodiazepines (Table 6.9), since the latter ones are thought to represent that part of GABA receptors connected with benzodiazepine receptors (see § 4.1.3).

On the other hand, despite this up-regulation of low- and high-affinity GABA receptors, GABA responsiveness seems to be decreased after chronic treatment with benzodiazepines, as has been found in electrophysiological experiments on neuronal sensitivity (Gallager *et al.*, 1984) and for the stimulatory effect of GABA on benzodiazepine receptor binding (Mele *et al.*, 1984) (see § 4.1.4). The biochemical basis of this phenomenon has not yet been elucidated.

6.4.2 *Relationship to functional tolerance and dependence*

Functional tolerance after chronic treatment with benzodiazepine is well documented in animals (File, 1984) and man (Greenblatt & Shader, 1978) and represents a pharmacodynamic rather than a pharmacokinetic phenomenon (Greenblatt & Shader, 1978). It is more pronounced for the sedative–hypnotic and the anticonvulsive than for the anxiolytic properties. Although tolerance to the sedative effects is sometimes useful in clinical practice, e.g. when the drugs are used as daytime tranquillizers, tolerance to the anticonvulsive properties is a limiting factor for the usefulness of benzodiazepines as antiepileptic drugs. Accordingly, an exact knowledge about the mechanisms leading to tolerance would be very helpful for the development of benzodiazepine derivatives showing this phenomenon to a lesser degree. Consequently, some attempts have been made to correlate benzodiazepine receptor down-regulation with functional tolerance. However, since clinically relevant tolerance develops with the usual therapeutic doses but receptor tolerance only with very high doses, little evidence yet exists that functional tolerance to benzodiazepines can be explained on the basis of benzodiazepine receptor down-regulation (Rosenberg & Chiu, 1981, 1982*b*). Some speculations have been reported, though, between regional differences of benzodiazepine receptor down-regulation and differences in the development of tolerance seen for the different pharmacological properties of the benzodiazepines (Tietz *et al.*, 1986).

Some recent data suggest that functional tolerance might be explained by a less-effective coupling of the benzodiazepine receptor to the GABA receptor after chronic benzodiazepine treatment (Sher *et al.*, 1983: Mele *et al.*, 1984) or/and by the subsensitivity of the postsynaptic GABA responsiveness observed under these conditions (Gallager *et al.*, 1984;

Gonsalves & Gallager, 1985), but this hypothesis needs further experimental confirmation.

Possibly the most serious complication of the therapeutic use of the benzodiazepines is the development of physical dependence, leading to withdrawal phenomena after discontinuation of the benzodiazepine therapy after prolonged treatment not only with high doses but also with therapeutic doses of benzodiazepines (Tyrer *et al.*, 1983; Schöpf, 1983; Ashton, 1984). Withdrawal phenomena have also been reported quite recently after long-term treatment of experimental animals with relatively low doses of benzodiazepines, with the observation that this phenomenon is more common in dogs than in rats or mice (McNicholas *et al.*, 1985; Scherkl & Frey, 1986). While studies with the benzodiazepine receptor antagonist Ro 15–1788 have clearly established that the development of dependence and the presence of withdrawal phenomena after cessation of therapy or after acute treatment with Ro 15–1788 are associated with the chronic activation of the benzodiazepine receptor by benzodiazepine agonists, the molecular nature of this phenomenon has not yet been found (Cumin *et al.*, 1982; Lukas & Griffiths, 1982; Rosenberg & Chiu, 1982*a*; Lamb & Griffiths, 1985). It is not correlated to the reduced number of benzodiazepine receptors (see above). Moreover, some recent studies suggest that the development of physical dependence with the presence of withdrawal phenomena after abrupt drug discontinuation is also not correlated to the development of tolerance for the effects of benzodiazepine agonist (Gonsalves & Gallager, 1985; Lamb & Griffiths, 1985).

In conclusion, at present we have little evidence that the down-regulation of benzodiazepine receptor density observed after chronic treatment with high doses of benzodiazepines is directly involved in the clinically important phenomena of tolerance and physical dependence.

6.4.3 *Chronic treatment with benzodiazepine receptor antagonists*

Chronic treatment with the two benzodiazepine receptor antagonists Ro 15–1788 and β-ECC produced up-regulation of benzodiazepine receptor density in several regions of the rat brain (Table 6.7). While β-ECC has some inverse agonistic properties, Ro 15–1788 is a rather 'pure' benzodiazepine receptor antagonist with few benzodiazepine-like agonistic properties. Accordingly, the similar findings for both antagonists cannot be explained on the basis of their slight intrinsic activities (which are different), but could be interpreted as a typical example of supersensitivity often seen after chronic treatment with receptor antagonists (Schweitzer *et al.*, 1984). This, however, requires the assumption that antagonist treatment chronically prevents the interaction of an endogenous benzodiazepine-like agonist with the receptor.

In conclusion, the data reported so far for the effects of chronic treatment with agonists and antagonists are compatible with the assumption of sub- or super-sensitivity of the benzodiazepine receptor, with the benzodiazepines mimicking the effect of a putative endogenous agonist.

6.4.4 *Denervation supersensitivity*

It seems to be a general physiological mechanism that the sensitivity of neuronal receptors increases when the supply of the neurotransmitter is reduced by interruption of afferents. Accordingly, the denervation of the inhibitory striatonigral GABAergic pathway, induced by the intrastriatal injection of kainic acid, has been demonstrated to result in an increase of the number of GABA receptors in the substantia nigra with no apparent change of the dissociation constant (Waddington & Cross, 1978). Moreover, GABA receptors of the substantia nigra become supersensitive for GABA-stimulated benzodiazepine receptor binding after these lesions (Shibuya *et al.*, 1980). The same procedure did not alter the number of benzodiazepine receptors in the substantia nigra, but reduced their affinity, probably by a reduction of the endogenous levels of GABA (Biggio *et al.*, 1979). Again, neuronal mechanisms regulating benzodiazepine receptor and GABA receptor levels are not identical. On the other hand, when similar lesions in the striatum were performed in rats which had received kainic acid injections in the substantia nigra, a pronounced increase of the density of benzodiazepine receptor was found in the substantia nigra relative to controls (having injections in the substantia nigra only) (Biggio *et al.*, 1981*a*). This increase is almost entirely due to an increase of the BZ_2 benzodiazepine receptor subclass (Porceddu *et al.*, 1985). These findings have been interpreted to mean that, for the development of denervation supersensitivity of benzodiazepine receptors, intrinsic neurons of the substantia nigra must also be destroyed and that at least the BZ_2 receptors are physiologically innervated by an endogenous ligand whose supply is interrupted by the lesions.

Dark-adaptation of rats has been reported to increase the density of benzodiazepine receptors in the retina, which also can be considered as evidence for denervation supersensitivity or, better, for supersensitivity after deprivation of the sensory input into this region of the CNS (Biggio *et al.*, 1981*b*; Rothe *et al.*, 1985).

Both examples suggest that denervation supersensitivity of benzodiazepine receptors can occur and is difficult to explain if one does not assume the presence of an endogenous agonist, whose interaction with the benzodiazepine receptor is interrupted by the lesions.

6.4.5 *Acute treatment with benzodiazepines*

No consistent data are available about the possible effect of an acute treatment with benzodiazepine agonists on the density of benzodiazepine receptors. Increased or decreased densities have been reported (Speth *et al.*, 1979; Coupet *et al.*, 1981). At present, most evidence indicates that these findings are not related to physiologically relevant sub- or super-sensitivity, but are artefacts due to a different solubility of the benzodiazepine receptor out of the neuronal membrane without or in the presence of benzodiazepine derivatives (Coupet *et al.*, 1981; Korneyev & Factor, 1981).

6.5 Summary

Unfortunately, none of the four experimental approaches has given an unequivocal answer to the question about the physiological function of the benzodiazepine receptor and about its putative ligand. Taking all the pieces of evidence together (see above), the puzzle is far from complete, but the picture now emerging is more in favour of a physiological function than not. However, even if we agree on that, we have to accept that this system is not very active under normal physiological conditions in animals or man, or alternatively, that its activity is not very relevant for the overall function of our CNS. This conclusion is strongly supported by the findings that the relatively pure benzodiazepine receptor antagonist Ro 15–1788 is, under most conditions, pharmacologically not or only very slightly active. On the other hand, the putative endogenous function of the benzodiazepine receptor system might become functionally relevant under certain specific conditions, e.g. when GABAergic transmission is experimentally (see § 6.2.2) or pathologically (see § 6.2.4) impaired. This might suggest that the benzodiazepine receptor system is not one of the major neuronal systems regulating CNS function, but rather that it represents some kind of auxiliary system, either to handle CNS function when other major neuronal systems fail, or to function as a certain kind of fine adjustment for some specific brain functions. Benzodiazepine drugs acting as a system for fine adjustment would also explain why benzodiazepines never depress CNS function as strongly as drugs like the barbiturates, which directly activate one of the major mechanisms to reduce neuronal excitability (see § 4.2).

In conclusion, it seems that the putative physiological role of the benzodiazepine receptor system is that of an auxiliary system to handle some specific effects or certain pathological situations. If this system is physiologically modulated in relation to over- or under-activity of the CNS, then it is most likely under conditions when it is functionally relevant, e.g. during pathological changes of CNS function. Accordingly, Chapter 7 reviews our present knowledge about pathological changes of the benzodiazepine receptor system in animals and man. Special emphasis will be placed on the question of how far these pathological changes support the putative endogenous function of the benzodiazepine receptor.

7

Pathological changes of the benzodiazepine receptor in animals and man

This chapter is closely related to the preceding one as it also deals with the possible physiological function of the benzodiazepine receptor. It specifically summarizes alterations of the properties of the benzodiazepine receptor under various pathological conditions in animals and man, and discusses the possible functional significance of the altered receptor properties. It is obvious that any defect at the benzodiazepine receptor system which seriously affects CNS function will represent an important link to the still-unknown physiological role of the benzodiazepine receptor.

7.1 Genetically determined changes in animals

Genetically determined alterations of the properties of the benzodiazepine receptor have been observed in a variety of neurologically mutant animals. These findings can be divided into two large categories, the first one including animals with known histological lesions, and the second one including animals for which histological abnormalities have not been found. The reasons for this split are easily explained. In mutants with well-known histological lesions, any change of the density of a given receptor system will very likely represent an effect of the histological lesion *per se*. Thus, such animals will give valuable information about the localization of a given receptor system rather than about its specific function. On the other hand, if histological lesions are not known, specific biochemical abnormalities of the mutant animals might represent important links to the nature of their neurological defects.

7.1.1 *Neurologically mutant animals with known histological lesions*

Most of the data summarized in this section refer to genetically determined abnormalities in the cerebellum, which represents a highly ordered structure with a limited number of different types of neuron. Since most of the neurological mouse mutants described in this section are characterized by a specific loss of one or more of the neuronal cell types of the cerebellum, receptor binding studies using these mutants are usually employed to investigate the localization of a given receptor at the different cell types of the mouse cerebellum.

Strong evidence for a location of benzodiazepine receptors on cerebellar Purkinje cells has been found in studies on the *nervous* and the *pcd* mutant mouse. The *nervous* mutant is characterized by a loss of about 90% of the cerebellar Purkinje cells, which results in a reduction of the benzodiazepine receptor density (in relation to mg membrane protein) by about 30% (Skolnick *et al.*, 1978*b*) or by about 80% (Lippa *et al.*, 1978). Similar findings (a reduction of receptor density by about 25%) have been reported for the *pcd* mouse at about 45 days of age, when cerebellar Purkinje cells are reduced by about 95% (Vaccarino *et al.*, 1983). Moreover, when the reduction of the number of benzodiazepine receptors was calculated on the basis of receptors per cerebellum, the reduction amounted to about 50% at an age of 45 days (Vaccarino *et al.*, 1983, 1985). Similar findings (a reduction of the number of receptors per cerebellum by about 90%) have been reported for the *Lurcher* mutant (Sauer *et al.*, 1984), which is characterized by an almost complete loss of cerebellar Purkinje cells and a 90% reduction of granule cells. On the other hand, the density of the benzodiazepine receptor seems to be unchanged or even elevated in the *Weaver* mutant (characterized by a nearly complete loss of granule cells) (Chang *et al.*, 1980). Accordingly, the findings about the largely decreased benzodiazepine receptor density in the *Lurcher* mutant (Sauer *et al.*, 1984) have been interpreted as strong evidence that the majority of cerebellar benzodiazepine receptors reside on Purkinje cells. These conclusions have been recently questioned on the basis of autoradiographic studies in the *Lurcher* cerebellum indicating no change of density relative to controls (Biscoe & Fry, 1984). However, since autoradiographic experiments reveal only receptor densities, these data do not exclude the possibility that the number of receptors calculated per cerebellum is largely decreased.

A reduced number of benzodiazepine receptors has been found in the spinal cord of the *sprawling* mouse, characterized by a deficiency of large-diameter myelinated axons of peripheral nerves and of the sensory roots and dorsal columns of the spinal cord. These findings have been interpreted as evidence for a presynaptic location of benzodiazepine receptors at primary afferent terminals (Biscoe & Fry, 1984).

Binding studies reported for the *jimpy* and the *dystrophic* mouse mutants suggest that benzodiazepine receptors do not reside on oligodendroglia or on peripheral nerves, which is in agreement with a variety of other studies using other approaches (Biscoe & Fry, 1984).

In conclusion, studies on neurologically mutant mice have given valuable information about the possible location of benzodiazepine receptors in the CNS.

7.1.2 *Neurologically mutant animals without known histological lesions*

As already mentioned, if histological abnormalities are not known, any biochemical abnormalities in such mutant animals can be much more closely related to neurological defects than is possible in the case of mutants with known histological lesions, where the most likely explanation for the biochemical abnormality is the histological lesion *per se*.

Good examples of such an approach are studies on the properties of the benzodiazepine receptor in the CNS of the mouse mutant *spastic* (White & Heller, 1982; Biscoe *et al.*, 1984). In both studies, the spinal cord of the *spastic* mouse was reported to have an increased number of benzodiazepine receptors, which has been interpreted as one of the compensatory mechanisms taking place to counterbalance the primary defect which is possibly located within the glycinergic neurotransmission. A similar 'up-regulation' of the GABA receptor has also been reported, so that the physiological relevance of the elevated number of benzodiazepine receptors is not yet finally known (White & Heller, 1982).

The mouse mutant *trembler* is characterized by an action-tremor which is absent if the animal is at rest. A large increase in the number of benzodiazepine receptors has been found in the forebrain of the *trembler* mouse when compared with littermate controls (Nunn *et al.*, 1983). It is not yet known whether this alteration itself represents one of the inherited lesions, or whether this defect is a secondary response again to counterbalance some other neurochemical defects in the CNS of the mouse mutant *trembler*. In both cases, the benzodiazepine receptors seem to have a physiologically relevant function. Thus, it might be important to investigate further the neurochemical defects of this mutant.

7.1.3 *Animals with a genetically determined susceptibility for audiogenic seizures*

Animals with a genetically determined susceptibility for epileptiform seizures represent important models in which to study the neurochemical basis of seizure disorders in man (Tacke & Braestrup, 1984), beside their use as animal models to test for anticonvulsive drugs. Accordingly, findings about changes of the properties of the benzodiazepine receptor in such animals might represent possible clues as to the nature of pathological defects of the benzodiazepine receptor present in various seizure disorders in man (Spero, 1982).

This approach was strongly supported by the findings of Robertson (1980), who found an elevated density of benzodiazepine receptors in an audiogenic seizure-susceptible strain of mouse when compared with a seizure-resistant strain. This difference was present only at the time of the sensitivity of the mice to the audiogenic seizures, since both phenomena (seizure-susceptibility and increased number of benzodiazepine receptors) disappeared when the mice became older (Robertson, 1980). These findings could not be reproduced by Horton *et al.* (1982), who did not find any relevant difference in the benzodiazepine receptor levels between seizure-susceptible and seizure-resistant mice. However, the authors found differences in the coupling mechanism between the GABA receptor and the benzodiazepine receptor, with an increased stimulation of benzodiazepine receptor binding by GABA at that time in the mice's lives when the seizure-susceptibility was maximal (Horton *et al.*, 1982). These findings could not be reproduced in a study using audiogenic seizure-susceptible rats, where a reduced stimulation of benzodiazepine receptor binding by the GABAergic agonist muscimol was found (Tacke & Braestrup, 1984). Again, no major changes in the properties of the benzodiazepine receptor itself were observed. Similarly, no differences of basal benzodiazepine receptor binding and GABA-stimulated benzodiazepine receptor binding have been found between control animals and seizure-susceptible epileptic fowl (Fisher *et al.*, 1985) or seizure-susceptible *El* mice (Hattori *et al.*, 1985).

On the other hand, a reduced benzodiazepine receptor density relative to controls has been found in some midbrain regions (substantia nigra, periaqueductal grey matter) of a seizure-susceptible gerbil (Olsen *et al.*, 1985), although the effects were paralleled by similar changes in low-affinity GABA receptors.

The interpretation of these findings is difficult, but it seems that changes in the properties of the benzodiazepine receptor are not a general aetiological factor for the increased seizure-susceptibility of these inbred animal strains. On the other hand, in most of these studies, differences in the benzodiazepine receptor system were reported for the seizure-susceptible animals, although these changes were quite different in each of the studies. Thus, it might be possible that changes at the benzodiazepine receptor level occur secondarily to the genetically determined increased seizure-susceptibility and represent adaptive changes of the brain, possibly to control the reduced seizure threshold. If we accept that these animal models are of some heuristic value to explain the biochemical basis of seizure disorders in man, the data would suggest that the major pathological defect of these disorders is not at the level of the benzodiazepine receptor. Indeed, this conclusion agrees with the data obtained for benzodiazepine receptor binding in *post mortem* brain samples of epileptic patients (see § 7.3.2).

7.1.4 *Animals with genetically determined different levels of emotionality*

Some experimental evidence suggests that changes in the benzodiazepine receptor might be involved in the relative level of emotionality of rats and mice. Since emotionality has usually been quantified in behavioural paradigms indicating anxiety, these data have been considered as indicative for a more-or-less direct relationship between the properties of the benzodiazepine receptor in several animal strains and their individual level of anxiety.

The first data were published by Robertson *et al.* (1978), who found that, within two strains of rats bred for high or low fearfulness, the latter had a significantly higher density of benzodiazepine receptors in several brain regions, especially the hippocampus and the hypothalamus. Comparable data were reported for an emotional strain of mouse which exhibited a higher density of benzodiazepine receptors in whole-brain homogenates than three non-emotional strains (Robertson, 1979), and for Roman high-avoidance and Roman low-avoidance rats with an increased density of benzodiazepine receptors in the first group (Gentsch *et al.*, 1981). Somewhat different data have been reported by Shephard *et al.* (1982), who found significantly elevated benzodiazepine receptor levels in Roman rats with either very high or very low levels of emotionality when compared with rats of intermediate emotionality. One of the possible explanations for these differences could be the use of different indices for measuring emotionality (active versus passive avoidance). On the other hand, the latter negative findings have been further substantiated recently by the failure to find any relationship between the level of benzodiazepine receptors and the level of emotionality for 18 different genotypes derived from Roman rats (Shephard *et al.*, 1984).

At present, it is not possible to draw a final conclusion from the data reported. Although the differences in benzodiazepine receptor binding between animal strains of different emotionality are in some cases present, final evidence is missing that the receptor changes *per se* are involved in the different emotionality. Again, it is possible that the receptor changes take place secondarily to the genetically determined different levels of emotionality and represent some kind of adaptive change.

7.1.5 *Summary*

As we have seen, changes of the properties of the benzodiazepine receptor seem to be present in the brains of various animals with genetically determined disorders of the CNS. However, the functional relevance of the alterations at the benzodiazepine receptor level is not yet known. Obviously, the earlier assumption that the density of benzodiazepine receptors could be directly correlated with pathological changes in brain function is not the case, and possibly was much too naive. The latter point is supported by recent animal data indicating no general correlation between receptor levels and function for benzodiazepines. Shephard *et al.* (1984) could not find a correlation between the benzodiazepine receptor levels of 18 genotypes derived from the Roman rat and their sensitivity for the benzodiazepine derivative diazepam (hyponeophagia test). Similar observations were made in five mouse strains, where the increase of the exploratory behaviour induced by diazepam did not correlate with the benzodiazepine receptor densities (Crawley & Davis, 1982), and in rats responding differently to benzodiazepines in an anticonflict test without exhibiting different levels of benzodiazepine receptors in three brain regions (Patel *et al.*, 1984). The most likely explanation for these observations is given by the findings that only a very small amount of the benzodiazepine receptor needs to be occupied to elicit a pharmacological response to a benzodiazepine (Braestrup *et al.*, 1983*b*). This huge number of 'spare' receptors explains that small variations in the concentration of benzodiazepine receptors are probably not always relevant to CNS function (see § 3.2). These considerations have to be taken into account in any attempt to correlate pathological changes of brain function with changed levels of benzodiazepine receptors and will also have important implications for studies on the properties of the benzodiazepine receptor in *post mortem* samples of pathological human brain. On the other hand, the findings that changes in the properties of the benzodiazepine receptor are sometimes present in these genetic animal models – where it is less important if the adaptive changes are relevant for the functional defect – strongly indicate a pronounced plasticity of this receptor system. Again, it is hard to understand why the brain should regulate this receptor in response to several dysfunctions if it has no use for it.

7.2 Pathological changes in animals

As outlined above, genetically determined lesions of brain function in animals lead to adaptive changes of the benzodiazepine receptor, rather than these changes representing inherited defects *per se*. This, however, makes it very likely that other CNS dysfunctions are also accompanied by similar adaptive changes of this receptor system. Again, the presence of specific adaptive changes of the benzodiazepine receptor in response to a given pathological defect of the CNS will give further evidence for a physiological role of this system.

7.2.1 *Effects of acute and chronic convulsions*

One of the most prominent pharmacological and clinical properties of the benzodiazepines is their effectiveness against convulsions. Accordingly, it is tempting to speculate that, if such adaptive changes do occur, they most likely do so as a specific response to acute or chronic convulsive states in experimental animals or in patients. And, indeed, several authors have reported profound alterations of the properties of the benzodiazepine receptor as a consequence of acute or repeated convulsions in experimental animals.

A rapid increase of benzodiazepine receptor binding has been found as response to both chemically and electrically induced convulsions (Paul & Skolnick, 1978; Asano & Mizutani, 1980; Lal *et al.*, 1981; Syapin & Rickman, 1981). The molecular basis for this observation is not yet clear, since these changes have been explained by an increase in either the receptor density or the receptor affinity. Moreover, a more recent report by Bowdler & Green (1982) failed to find significant changes in benzodiazepine receptor binding after acute convulsions, but reported an increase of GABA levels in many brain regions after electrically induced convulsions. Thus, the rather inconsistent changes found by the other authors might represent indirect effects, caused by an increased benzodiazepine receptor affinity due to the elevated level of endogenously present GABA. This might also explain the pronounced inconsistency of the data reported (see above), since because of different washing procedures during the membrane preparation for the binding assays, levels of endogenous GABA and therefore *in vitro* GABA stimulation of benzodiazepine receptor binding might have been different.

Significant alterations of the density of benzodiazepine receptor have also been found after the administration of repeated seizures to experimental animals or after the related procedure of 'kindling', a progressive enhancement of stimulus-induced epileptiform activity, which represents an important animal model for epilepsy. It seems from the data available that these alterations exhibit a biphasic time course, with a profound increase in receptor density 24 h after the last seizure (McNamara *et al.*, 1980) which is followed by a long-lasting decrease of receptor density for more than 60 days in the cortex and hypothalamus, but not in the hippocampus (Burnham *et al.*, 1983; Niznik *et al.*, 1983). However, conflicting data to the latter findings have also been reported using a well-washed membrane preparation (Niznik *et al.*, 1984). This could indicate that kindling or related procedures do not down-regulate the density of the benzodiazepine receptor directly, but induce the long-lasting production of an endogenous factor which interferes with the experimental determination of benzodiazepine receptor density. This, however, is speculative. On the other hand, a similar phenomenon has already been found when a high concentration of a benzodiazepine derivative is present in a brain homogenate, which is used for the preparation of membrane fragments for the binding assay (Korneyev & Factor, 1981) (see § 6.4.5). A decrease in benzodiazepine receptors has also been found in the hippocampus after electrolytic lesions of the entorhinal cortex in the rat (Kraus *et al.*, 1983).

In conclusion, there is little conclusive evidence in favour of changes in the density of the benzodiazepine receptor representing a specific response to chronic or repeated seizures. On the other hand, such procedures might change the GABA levels in the CNS and thus alter endogenous GABA stimulation of benzodiazepine receptor binding (Niznik *et al.*, 1984). While this might account for some of the observations of altered benzodiazepine receptor binding, a full explanation for observations concerning changes of receptor density cannot yet been given. Although quite attractive, the hypothesis that changes of the benzodiazepine receptor are directly involved in the pathogenesis of 'epileptiform' disorders in animals currently receives little experimental support from the data reported.

not assume the presence of an endogenous agonist, whose interaction with the benzodiazepine receptor is interrupted by the lesions.

6.4.5 *Acute treatment with benzodiazepines*

No consistent data are available about the possible effect of an acute treatment with benzodiazepine agonists on the density of benzodiazepine receptors. Increased or decreased densities have been reported (Speth *et al.*, 1979; Coupet *et al.*, 1981). At present, most evidence indicates that these findings are not related to physiologically relevant sub- or super-sensitivity, but are artefacts due to a different solubility of the benzodiazepine receptor out of the neuronal membrane without or in the presence of benzodiazepine derivatives (Coupet *et al.*, 1981; Korneyev & Factor, 1981).

6.5 Summary

Unfortunately, none of the four experimental approaches has given an unequivocal answer to the question about the physiological function of the benzodiazepine receptor and about its putative ligand. Taking all the pieces of evidence together (see above), the puzzle is far from complete, but the picture now emerging is more in favour of a physiological function than not. However, even if we agree on that, we have to accept that this system is not very active under normal physiological conditions in animals or man, or alternatively, that its activity is not very relevant for the overall function of our CNS. This conclusion is strongly supported by the findings that the relatively pure benzodiazepine receptor antagonist Ro 15–1788 is, under most conditions, pharmacologically not or only very slightly active. On the other hand, the putative endogenous function of the benzodiazepine receptor system might become functionally relevant under certain specific conditions, e.g. when GABAergic transmission is experimentally (see § 6.2.2) or pathologically (see § 6.2.4) impaired. This might suggest that the benzodiazepine receptor system is not one of the major neuronal systems regulating CNS function, but rather that it represents some kind of auxiliary system, either to handle CNS function when other major neuronal systems fail, or to function as a certain kind of fine adjustment for some specific brain functions. Benzodiazepine drugs acting as a system for fine adjustment would also explain why benzodiazepines never depress CNS function as strongly as drugs like the barbiturates, which directly activate one of the major mechanisms to reduce neuronal excitability (see § 4.2).

animals, a clear impression of a specific and predictable change has not yet emerged.

7.2.3 *Effect of stress and benzodiazepine receptor ligands on GABA receptor binding*

As outlined above, there is little final evidence for an up- or down-regulation of benzodiazepine receptors as a general feature of experimental stress. Biggio *et al.* (1984) have presented another hypothesis concerning a possible benzodiazepine receptor-related mechanism involved in the central regulation of stress, which includes the modulation of low-affinity GABA receptor properties by benzodiazepine receptor ligands. Biggio and his colleagues found that acute stress (handling of rats before killing by guillotine) decreased the density of cortical low-affinity GABA receptors relative to control animals habituated to the handling procedure over a period of 10 days. The decrease of cortical low-affinity GABA receptors was of a similar degree to that observed after the *in vitro* addition of inverse benzodiazepine receptor agonists (β-carbolines) to cortical membranes of habituated rats (Concas *et al.*, 1985*a*). Both stress-induced and β-carboline-induced reduction of GABA receptor density could be antagonized by the agonist diazepam as well as by the pure antagonist Ro 15–1788. Biggio *et al.* (1984) interpreted their data by suggesting that stress releases an endogenous compound which down-regulates GABA receptors by interacting with the benzodiazepine receptor in a manner similar to inverse agonists. It is important to note that only the low-affinity GABA receptors were changed after these manipulations, since some evidence exists that the low-affinity GABA receptors are specifically connected with the benzodiazepine receptor (see § 4.1.3).

Similar findings were reported by the same authors about the effects of electrical foot shock on the density of cortical low-affinity GABA receptors (Concas *et al.*, 1985*b*), which could also be prevented by the *in vivo* administration of the specific benzodiazepine receptor antagonist Ro 15–1788 prior to the foot shock procedure.

These findings, which suggest the presence of an endogenous inverse agonist of the benzodiazepine receptor which regulates GABA receptor function in relation to stress, anxiety and fear, seem very attractive, but further experimental support is needed.

7.2.4 *Effect of gender and sex hormones*

Several lines of evidence suggest that emotionality differs between male and female mammals, including man, and that sex hormones might play a role in regulating the different levels of emotionality (Gray, 1971; Donovan, 1985). Assuming that differences at the level of the benzodiazepine receptor could account at least partially for these sex differences, Shephard *et al.* (1982) investigated the density of benzodiazepine receptors in various brain regions of male and female Roman rats. Higher receptor densities for the male animals were found in the hippocampus and the striatum, while higher densities for the female animals were present in the cortex and the cerebellum. Similar findings have been reported in the mouse, with a higher density of the benzodiazepine receptor in the female than in the male mouse brain (Sonawane *et al.*, 1980).

The functional significance of these findings is not yet known, but recent data suggest that they might have an endocrine basis. While chronic treatment with oestradiol for 1 month did not alter benzodiazepine receptor densities in native female rats (Goetz *et al.*, 1983), long-term treatment of ovariectomized rats with oestradiol for 3 months resulted in a significant increase in benzodiazepine receptor density in the hypothalamus when compared with untreated but ovariectomized animals (Wilkinson *et al.*, 1983). Similar observations were made with native rats and mice treated with very high doses of oestradiol (Wilkinson *et al.*, 1983). An increase in benzodiazepine receptor density in the cerebellum was also found in ovariectomized rats after treatment with oestradiol, while GABA receptor binding was elevated in the same animals in the caudate, the frontal cortex, the hippocampus and the olfactory bulb (Maggi *et al.*, 1984). Treatment with progesterone affected GABA receptor binding in the caudate and the frontal cortex, but did not affect benzodiazepine receptor binding (Maggi *et al.*, 1984). When male rats were treated with oestradiol, GABA receptor binding was elevated in the cortex and benzodiazepine receptor binding in the cerebellum (Maggi *et al.*, 1984).

These data suggest that the endocrine status of rats and mice might be one of the physiological factors regulating the benzodiazepine receptor system and its putative endogenous function (Shephard *et al.*, 1982).

7.2.5 *Changes in thyroid state*

The properties of the benzodiazepine receptor can be dramatically altered by different thyroid states in rats, with a 25% decrease in receptor density in rats rendered hyperthyroid by chronic treatment with *L*-triiodothyronine, and a 40% increase in receptor density in rats rendered hypothyroid by thyroidectomy (Medina & De Robertis, 1985). In both cases, the affinity of the receptor for benzodiazepines was unchanged, but the affinity of the thyroid hormone triiodothyronine was nearly two orders of magnitude higher in hypo- than in hyper-thyroid rats. Although these data are in line with the assumption of sub- or super-sensitivity of the benzodiazepine receptor in relation to the brain levels of thyroid hormones as putative endogenous ligands (§ 6.1.3), I think that the brain levels of these hormones are still much too low to support this assumption. It seems much more likely that the thyroid status modulates benzodiazepine receptor properties via a different mechanism, possibly by changing the brain levels of another endogenous ligand or as an adaptive response to an altered brain function. The latter assumption is supported by findings about an unchanged seizure threshold for pentetrazole or bicuculline (drugs acting at the benzodiazepine receptor–GABA receptor complex) in rats rendered hyperthyroid by chronic treatment with triiodothyronine (Atterwill & Nutt, 1983). These findings would suggest that, although the density of the benzodiazepine receptors is reduced in this state, the final function of the benzodiazepine receptor–GABA receptor complex is unaltered.

To what extent similar adaptive changes of the benzodiazepine receptor during pathological thyroid states are present in man and might be relevant for some of the CNS disturbances frequently seen in patients with thyroid disease is not yet known. Data on benzodiazepine receptor properties in *post mortem* brain samples of patients with thyroid disease have not yet been reported. On the other hand, recently published data on experimentally induced hyper- as well as hypo-thyroid states in experimental animals suggest that alterations at the level of the benzodiazepine receptor are not a specific response of thyroid disease, since the properties of dopamine, muscarinic and GABA receptors are changed as well (Kalaria & Prince, 1986).

7.2.6 *Changes with age*

Several experimental and clinical observations indicate that sensitivity for benzodiazepines increases in man with age, an effect which can be explained only partially by age-related changes in pharmacokinetics (Klotz, 1984). Accordingly, age-related changes in the benzodiazepine receptor could represent an additional explanation. However, totally conflicting data have been reported about age-related changes of benzodiazepine receptor density in experimental animals: no change (Pedigo *et al.*, 1981; Tsang *et al.*, 1982), an increase (hippocampus only)

(Memo *et al.*, 1981), and a decrease (hippocampus and cortex) (De Blasi *et al.*, 1982) have been found for rats of different strains (Fischer 344 or Sprague-Dawley). Although a final interpretation of these data is difficult, it seems that age-related hypersensitivity for benzodiazepines cannot be explained on the basis of changes in the benzodiazepine receptor in the aged brain.

Very interesting, but still very speculative findings have recently been reported by Reeves & Schweitzer (1983), who found differences in the relative increase of BZ_1 and BZ_2 benzodiazepine receptors after an acute treatment with diazepam between young and aged Fischer 344 rats, while the baseline levels of the two receptor subclasses were similar in both groups. Moreover, the different ontogenesis of the two receptor subclasses has been made responsible for paradoxical responses of immature rats to benzodiazepines (Barr & Lithgow, 1983). However, it is too early to draw any final conclusions from these findings with respect to their possible relevance for the age-related supersensitivity of animals and man for benzodiazepines.

7.2.7 *Summary*

The present review of pathological changes of the benzodiazepine receptor in experimental animals again demonstrates the profound plasticity of the system as indicated by the multiplicity of changes seen. However, if one goes very critically over all the existing data, there is little evidence to suggest that the changes at the benzodiazepine receptor level are directly relevant to the pathological state of the animals. In other words, pathological symptoms are probably not caused by alterations of the benzodiazepine receptor. Again, the impression emerges that the differences observed represent adaptive changes of the CNS in response to different pathological states. And again the question emerges, why should the brain modulate this receptor system if it has no use for it? In this respect it is important to note that, in most of the alterations reported, the benzodiazepine receptor was regulated independently of the GABA receptor.

7.3 Pathological changes in man

If one considers the efficiency of the benzodiazepines in treating anxiety states, sleep disorders, convulsive states and muscle spasms, it is very tempting to speculate that dysfunctions at the benzodiazepine receptor as the primary locus of benzodiazepine action are involved in the aetiology of these disorders. Accordingly, several attempts have been made to identify alterations at the benzodiazepine receptor system in the course of many neuropsychiatric disorders. A review of these data is given in this section. Since, in most cases, the aetiology of the disease is unknown, no attempt has been made to divide the data into genetically determined and presumably pathologically determined alterations, as was done for the animal data. The animal data have shown that this split is not very useful since, even in genetically determined lesions of the animals, most changes at the benzodiazepines receptor level were secondary to the primary (genetically determined) defect. Most of the studies reviewed have focused on changes in the density of the benzodiazepine receptor in various human brain areas. These data are summarized in Tables 7.1 and 7.2, where relevant findings with regard to other parameters of the benzodiazepine receptor system have been made, e.g. changes in the receptor affinity or in the coupling mechanism with the GABA receptor. These will be referred to in the text.

7.3.1 *Mental disorders (see Table 7.1)*

As indicated by the data from two studies, no evidence is present for an alteration in the benzodiazepine receptor in several brain areas of schizophrenics. As far as it has been investigated, GABA binding is also not changed, e.g. in the nucleus caudatus and the putamen (Owen *et al.*, 1981) and the frontal cortex (Bennett *et al.*, 1979) of schizophrenic patients.

Similar negative findings have been reported for two regions of human brain in depression. In the same study, no changes in GABA receptor binding were reported for one cortical area (Crow *et al.*, 1984). In contrast to these findings is the recent report by Cheetham *et al.* (1985) indicating an elevated density (+19%) of benzodiazepine receptors in the frontal but not the temporal cortex of 11 suicide victims with a firm diagnosis of depression. GABA receptor function, as measured by the $GABA_A$ receptor-mediated increase of benzodiazepine receptor binding by GABA, was not changed. No interpretation of these conflicting data is yet possible, but further studies on possible changes of the benzodiazepine receptor in depression are certainly desirable.

Cortical benzodiazepine receptors also are unaltered in alcoholics, in contrast to the elevation of GABA receptors in the same brain samples (Tran *et al.*, 1980). These findings have been interpreted as a supersensitivity of GABA receptors in response to a decreased level of GABA in the brain of alcoholics (Tran *et al.*, 1980). The up-regulation of the GABA receptor was not accompanied by a parallel change in the benzodiazepine receptor, indicating that independent regulation of the two receptor systems also takes place in human brain.

One early report of a slight increase in benzodiazepine receptor density in senile dementia of the Alzheimer type could not be confirmed in a later report of the same group. Accordingly, there is little evidence for a specific alteration of the benzodiazepine receptor in this disease.

Recent data indicate that the level of the benzodiazepine receptor is also not changed in four areas of human brain in Lesch–Nyhan syndrome.

Table 7.1 *Pathological changes in human brain: I. Mental disorders*

Changes in the density of the benzodiazepine receptor (B_{max}) in *post mortem* brain samples of patients suffering from different mental disorders. Changes of B_{max} are calculated in relation to control data (brain samples of patients without mental disorders).

Disease	Brain region	% change of B_{max}	Reference
Schizophrenia	Frontal cortex	±0	Reisine *et al.*
	Putamen	±0	(1980*b*)
	Nucleus caudatus	±0	
	Putamen	±0	Owen *et al.*
	Nucleus caudatus	±0	(1981)
Depression	Frontal cortex	±0	Crow *et al.*
	Hippocampus	±0	(1984)
	Frontal cortex	+19	Cheetham *et al.*
	Temporal cortex	±0	(1985)
Alcoholism	Frontal cortex	±0	Tran *et al.* (1980)
Senile dementia Alzheimer type	Temporal cortex	+13	Owen *et al.* (1983)
	Frontal cortex	±0	Crow *et al.*
	Temporal cortex	±0	(1984)
	Hippocampus	±0	
Lesch–Nyhan syndrome	Occipital cortex	±0	Kish *et al.*
	Temporal cortex	±0	(1985*a*)
	Frontal cortex	±0	
	Parietal cortex	±0	

This syndrome is associated with a severe neurological disorder characterized by choreioform and athetoid movements, hypertonicity, mental retardation and self-injurious behaviour. Its biochemical defect is an inherited and complete deficiency of the enzyme hypoxanthine–guanine phosphoribosyltransferase. This finally leads to a pronounced dysfunction of dopaminergic neurons, which might explain same of the neurological symptoms (Baumeister & Frye, 1984; Silverstein *et al.*, 1985). On the other hand, due to the primary defect within the purine metabolism, the purines inosine and hypoxanthine are markedly elevated in the cerebrospinal fluid and in *post mortem* brain samples of patients with Lesch–Nyhan syndrome (Kish *et al.*, 1985*a*). These observations make this syndrome important for benzodiazepine receptor research, since inosine and hypoxanthine have been proposed as candidates for the endogenous ligand of the benzodiazepine receptor (see § 6.1.2). If this were the case, an increased level of both putative endogenous ligands should result in a down-regulation of the benzodiazepine receptor, which has not been observed. Thus, the unchanged level of the benzodiazepine receptor in this disease supports the general doubts about a physiological role of the two purines as benzodiazepine receptor ligands. On the other hand, GABA stimulation of benzodiazepine receptor binding was markedly reduced and the affinity of hypoxanthine for the benzodiazepine receptor was slightly increased in the cortex of Lesch–Nyhan patients. These observations might contribute to some of the neurological symptoms of this syndrome, but certainly do not represent the major biochemical lesion in Lesch–Nyhan syndrome (Kish *et al.*, 1985*a*).

Using positron emission tomography and [^{11}C]Ro 15–1788 as radioligand, Persson *et al.* (1985) found some evidence of an increased density of benzodiazepine receptors in several brain regions of two psychiatric patients who had been treated with high doses of benzodiazepines for many years to alleviate an incapacitating anxiety syndrome (about 80–100 mg diazepam per day). These preliminary data have to be interpreted very carefully, and two explanations are possible. The first would be to assume a benzodiazepine receptor up-regulation, as has been seen in experimental animals after prolonged treatment with very high doses (see § 6.4.1). The second would be to assume an elevated density of benzodiazepine receptors due to the chronic anxiety syndrome. The limited data available at present make a final decision as to which of the two assumptions is correct impossible. Nevertheless, these preliminary data indicate the usefulness of positron emission tomography for *in vivo* receptor visualization in the patient.

7.3.2 *Neurological disorders (see Table 7.2)*

As already outlined in § 7.1.3 about animal models of seizure disorders, it seems very likely that changes at the level of the benzodiazepine receptor level are present in epilepsy, either primarily as one of the aetiological factors or secondarily as an adaptive response to the decreased seizure threshold (Spero, 1982). Surprisingly, the only report so far about the properties of the benzodiazepine receptor system in *post mortem* brain samples of epileptic patients indicates not only no changes in the benzodiazepine receptor density, but also no changes in GABA receptor

Table 7.2 *Pathological changes in human brain: II. Neurological disorders*

Changes in the density of the benzodiazepine receptor (B_{max}) in *post mortem* brain samples of patients suffering from different neurological disorders. Changes of B_{max} are calculated in relation to control data (brain samples of patients without neurological disorders).

Disease	Brain region	% change of B_{max}	Reference
Epilepsy	Nucleus caudatus Hippocampus Frontal cortex Temporal cortex	±0 ±0 ±0 ±0	Wusteman *et al.* (1985)
Chorea Huntington	Frontal cortex Putamen Cerebellum	+27 −35 +32	Reisine *et al.* (1979)
	Putamen Substantia nigra	−33 +20	Reisine *et al.* (1980*a*)
	Putamen Lat. globus pallidus	−50 +40	Penney & Young (1982)
	Cerebellum	±0	Kish *et al.* (1983)
	Cortex Putamen Lat. globus pallidus Med. globus pallidus	±0 −56 +72 ±0	Walker *et al.* (1984)
Olivoponto-cerebellar atrophy	Cerebellar cortex	+29	Kish *et al.* (1984)
	Molecular layer Granule cell layer Dentate nucleus	±0 ±0 +150	Whitehouse *et al.* (1986)
Dialysis encephalopathy	Frontal cortex	−23	Kish *et al.* (1985*b*)

density and no changes of GABA stimulation of benzodiazepine receptor binding (Wusteman *et al.*, 1985). Although this is in agreement with some of the animal data (see § 7.1.3), the conclusion of a practically undisturbed benzodiazepine receptor–GABA receptor complex in epilepsy is still very unexpected, especially if one considers the pronounced plasticity of this receptor in experimental seizures in animals, not as an aetiological factor, but as an adaptive response (§ 7.2.1). Thus, the unchanged level in epileptic patients might have implications for understanding benzodiazepine receptor plasticity in man. Accordingly, more data are urgently needed.*

Several reports exist on alterations of benzodiazepine receptor levels in some brain regions of patients who died of Huntington's chorea. The most consistent observation is a reduced density in the putamen. Initial findings about an elevated level of benzodiazepine receptors in the cortex and the cerebellum could not be confirmed in later studies. More recent studies, however, indicate that the decrease in the receptor density in the striatum is accompanied by an increase of the density in the substantia nigra and the globus pallidus (Penney & Young, 1982; Walker *et al.*, 1984), two areas of the brain receiving neuronal input from the striatum. The decrease in the benzodiazepine receptor number in the striatum is usually explained by the neuronal loss in the striatum of Huntington's diseased patients and is paralleled by a similar decrease of some other neuroreceptors (Penney & Young, 1982; Walker *et al.*, 1984). Similar changes can be seen in rats after intrastriatal injections of kainic acid which destroys the cell bodies (Sperk & Schlögl, 1979) and which has been proposed as an animal model of this disease (Coyle & Schwarz, 1976). On the other hand, the recent studies by Walker *et al.* (1984) indicate that the loss of striatal benzodiazepine receptors precedes the degradation of striatal neurons, possibly indicating a preterminal dysfunction of these nerve cells. The subsequent increase in benzodiazepine receptors in the substantia nigra and the globus pallidus is paralleled by similar changes in the GABA receptor in both areas (Penney & Young, 1982; Walker *et al.*, 1984) and possibly represents denervation supersensitivity due to a loss of GABAergic projections from the striatum into both areas. In agreement with this assumption are the observations that GABA and benzodiazepine receptor densities increase in the substantia nigra of the rat after chemical lesions of the striatum (Biggio *et al.*, 1981*a*). Interestingly, GABA stimulation of benzodiazepine receptor binding is not different from controls in the

* A very recent report (Sherwin *et al.*, 1986) also indicates no changes of cortical benzodiazepine receptors in epileptic human brain.

putamen and the substantia nigra of Huntington's diseased patients (Reisine *et al.*, 1980*a*), indicating no defect of the coupling mechanism between the benzodiazepine and the GABA receptor. Up to now, the functional significance of the changes at the benzodiazepine receptor level in the course of Huntington's chorea is not known. However, these distinct and fairly well investigated changes might provide a good example of the complexity of biochemical changes at the neuroreceptor level which can take place during neuropsychiatric disorders.

An increase in the density of the benzodiazepine receptor in the cerebellar cortex has also been described for patients with olivopontocerebellar atrophy, a dominantly inherited cerebellar ataxia with a deficiency of cerebellar Purkinje cells (Table 7.2, see Kish *et al.*, 1984). This finding disagrees with observations in several animal mutants deficient in cerebellar Purkinje cells (see § 7.1.1), which usually exhibit a significant decrease of benzodiazepine receptor density in the cerebellum. The discrepancy cannot be explained entirely by the smaller level of benzodiazepine receptors on human than on rat or mouse Purkinje cells (Young & Kuhar, 1979), but rather suggests a compensatory mechanism, e.g. adaptive changes of benzodiazepine receptor density on neuronal elements of human cerebellum other than the Purkinje cells (Kish *et al.*, 1984). It should be added that the increase in benzodiazepine receptor density was most pronounced in only four of the patients investigated, all of the same pedigree (+77%). The increase of the benzodiazepine receptor was much less pronounced in all other patients, originating from different pedigrees (Kish *et al.*, 1984). The latter findings suggest the absence of a very close correlation between the symptoms of olivopontocerebellar atrophy and the increased level of cerebellar benzodiazepine receptors. These observations have been confirmed very recently, and the same authors (Whitehouse *et al.*, 1986) demonstrated that the increase in cerebellar benzodiazepine receptors was mainly in the dentate nucleus (Table 7.2). Since the dentate nucleus receives neuronal projections from the Purkinje cells (which are probably dysfunctional in this disease), the authors interpreted this observation as benzodiazepine receptor supersensitivity due to a loss of GABAergic projections from the Purkinje cells. Interestingly, GABA receptors as measured by [^{3}H]muscimol binding were not changed in the dentate nucleus of patients with olivopontocerebellar atrophy.

A reduced density of cortical benzodiazepine receptors has been found in patients who died from dialysis encephalopathy, a severe neurological disorder with seizures, speech abnormalities, progressive global dementia and psychotic episodes (Kish *et al.*, 1985*b*). The explanation for this observation is not yet known, especially since GABA receptor levels are unchanged in this disease while the GABA level in the brain is markedly reduced (Kish *et al.*, 1985*b*). Thus, GABAergic inhibition seems to be impaired in the brain of these patients and the expected compensatory change within the benzodiazepine receptor–GABA receptor system would be an increase of neuronal function rather than a decrease. To what extent the decrease in benzodiazepine receptors can be explained by a neuronal loss in the cortex of these patients needs further clarification.

In summary, although alterations at the benzodiazepine receptor level have been found in *post mortem* human brain samples in a variety of neuropsychiatric disorders, the aetiological role and the functional relevance of these alterations remain to be established.

7.4 Synopsis

The data reported and summarized in this chapter clearly show that the density of the benzodiazepine receptor is altered in the course of a variety of pathological states in animals and man. Since only a few of these findings can be explained by histological lesions of the neuronal structures where these receptors are localized, the data strongly indicate that the density of the benzodiazepine receptor *per se* is changed. Two major questions arise from these observations.

1 Are the pathological changes of the benzodiazepine receptor a phenomenon specific for this neuronal system?
2 Are the pathological changes of the benzodiazepine receptor part of the primary pathological defect or only a secondary adaptive response?

Taking the question of the specificity of the pathological changes of the benzodiazepine receptor, the most obvious argument against such a specificity would be the assumption that any change at the benzodiazepine receptor only mirrors a similar change of the postsynaptic part of the GABAergic synapse. In other words, changes of the benzodiazepine receptor would serve only as a marker for similar changes of the GABA receptor–benzodiazepine receptor complex, with the GABA receptor as the physiologically relevant part. Most of the available data speak very much against this assumption, since in many cases benzodiazepine receptor density changes without concomitant changes in the GABA receptor, and, even more important, in some cases GABA receptor properties are altered in a manner opposite to the properties of the benzodiazepine receptor. Thus, at least in some pathological conditions, specific changes of the benzodiazepine receptor *per se* take place. This observation might represent an important hint for a physiological role of this system. Why should the brain alter the properties of the benzodiazepine receptor if it has no use for it?

With regard to the second question, little evidence is present that the changes at the benzodiazepine receptor are primarily involved in the pathological conditions or are even responsible for some symptoms of the pathological conditions. This is the case for all animal data, where the pathological changes seem to be secondary to the primary lesion of the CNS and might represent adaptive responses of the CNS of these animals. In other words, the animals did not have CNS symptoms because of the change at the benzodiazepine receptor, but changed the benzodiazepine receptor properties as a response to disturbances of the CNS. This fits nicely into the theory that the benzodiazepine receptor system represents a neuronal system for 'fine adjustment' rather than for regulating the overall activity of central neurons. It seems conceivable that alterations of such a mechanism are very likely to occur in situations where the brain wants to counterbalance different pathological dysfunctions.

In view of the marked plasticity of the benzodiazepine receptor system during a variety of pathological states in animals, astonishingly few changes at the benzodiazepine receptor system have been found in samples of pathological human brain so far. While this might be less unexpected for the brains of depressive or schizophrenic patients, where benzodiazepines are not very effective in treating the primary disorder, the findings about unchanged properties of the benzodiazepine receptor in the brains of epileptic patients is certainly quite unexpected. This is in stark contrast to the animal data, where nearly any change of the seizure threshold profoundly alters the properties of the benzodiazepine receptor system, although the changes are not homogeneous for the different animal experiments. These findings cannot be explained with our present knowledge, but strongly suggest that the regulation or the plasticity of the benzodiazepine receptor in human brain differs considerably from that in the brain of experimental animals, although its molecular properties are very similar (Chapter 5). Thus, one has to be very careful in extrapolating animal data about benzodiazepine receptor plasticity to man. On the other hand, adaptive changes of the benzodiazepine receptor in response to pathologically disturbed brain functions do occur in human brain and might also give some hints for the physiological role of the benzodiazepine receptor in man.

8

Drug acceptor or physiological receptor?

8.1 Certainly a drug acceptor

As outlined in the previous chapters, overwhelming evidence has been presented over the last few years that the benzodiazepine receptor represents the locus of benzodiazepine action at the neuronal level in the CNS. These findings are valid not only for nearly all pharmacological properties in experimental animals, but also for all major clinical effects in man. They are supported by robust correlations between receptor affinity or receptor occupancy and *in vivo* potency, and by the presence of highly selective benzodiazepine receptor antagonists, able to terminate specifically practically all benzodiazepine effects in animals and man within a few minutes when given intravenously. Similarly strong evidence indicates that, by binding to this receptor, benzodiazepines or related drugs enhance the synaptic activity of the inhibitory neurotransmitter GABA by presumably allosteric mechanisms. These, however, are not yet very well understood. The final result at the electrophysiological level, though, is an increased frequency of single channel opening events in response to a given amount of synaptically released or exogenously applied GABA. Moreover, drugs like β-MCC, which also bind to the benzodiazepine receptor with high selectivity, show a pharmacological profile opposite to that of the benzodiazepines. Again, the primary locus of neuronal activity is the benzodiazepine receptor, but the electrophysiological correlate is a decrease of GABAergic neurotransmission due to a decreased frequency of single chloride channel opening events in response to GABA. Both types of pharmacological activity can be blocked by selective and competitive benzodiazepine receptor antagonists like Ro 15–1788. Thus, the benzodiazepine receptor represents at least a drug acceptor, with a pharmacological spectrum reaching from full agonist (benzodiazepines) over more or less pure antagonists (Ro 15–1788) to full inverse agonists (some β-carbolines).

Considering the highly differentiated properties of this receptor system, three questions again arise: why should our brains possess such a highly sophisticated binding site, why should evolution have produced such a specific system at the step from non-vertebrates to vertebrates, and why should evolution have maintained this specific system if there were no biological function or use for it? These and several other arguments (see below) strongly suggest to me that the presence of an endogenous ligand has to be assumed.

8.2 Also a receptor for a putative co-transmitter of GABAergic neurons?

The major aspects which support or argue against the putative physiological function of the benzodiazepine receptor can be summarized as follows.

1. An endogenous ligand of the benzodiazepine receptor has not yet been definitively identified. Certainly the most attractive candidate is DBI, but DBI probably functions only as a precursor molecule for one or more molecules of the putative ligand, which presumably represents a much smaller peptide. If we assume that the final ligand exhibits the same pharmacological properties as the precursor DBI, it represents an inverse agonist with proconvulsive and anxiogenic properties.
2. The presence of an anxiogenic (inverse agonistic) endogenous benzodiazepine receptor ligand is also supported by findings about Ro 15–1788-sensitive alterations of low-affinity GABA receptors by stress and electrical foot shock in rats.
3. The presence of an endogenous benzodiazepine receptor ligand with inverse agonistic properties is not supported by most studies on the possible effects of the pure antagonist Ro 15–1788 in animals or man, indicating the presence of an endogenous ligand with agonistic (benzodiazepine-like) rather than inverse agonistic properties.
4. All studies with the pure antagonist Ro 15–1788 have in common the observation of distinct but usually only very small effects, which seem to become more pronounced under conditions when GABAergic transmission is impaired in animals or man. Thus, the putative endogenous ligand might be of minor functional

relevance under normal conditions, but might become more relevant under certain pathological states.

5 The effects of chronic treatment with benzodiazepine receptor agonists and antagonists on benzodiazepine receptor density (down- and up-regulation) are consistent with the assumption of the presence of endogenous (benzodiazepine-like) agonists.

6 Several data in experimental animals and to a lesser extent in man indicate a pronounced plasticity of the benzodiazepine receptor system as a response to but not as the cause of various pathological states of the CNS. The modulation of benzodiazepine receptor properties is in some cases independent of adaptive changes of the GABA receptor and strongly suggests a physiological role of the benzodiazepine receptor itself.

If taken together, the data are very much in favour of a physiological role of the benzodiazepine receptor, although most evidence is still indirect. The observations of usually distinct but rather small effects mediated through the endogenous benzodiazepine receptor system agree with the biological findings indicating an auxiliary or fine-adjusting function of the benzodiazepine receptor system for inhibitory GABAergic neurotransmission. This fits nicely into the hypothesis that the putative endogenous ligand(s) is(are) co-released at GABAergic synapses, possibly from the same presynaptic neuron (Costa, 1983). Thus, it is very likely that the putative endogenous effector acts as a co-transmitter and not as the primary transmitter. The major difference is that only those signals that can be transduced are primary transmitters, whereas the co-transmitter operates on a mechanism that changes the efficacy of operation of the transducer (Costa *et al.*, 1984). In other words, only the receptor of the primary transmitter (GABA) is coupled to the transducer (chloride channel), while the receptor of the co-transmitter (benzodiazepine receptor) functions only as a modulatory unit of the coupling mechanism between the receptor of the primary transmitter and the transducer. This very attractive hypothesis goes in line with other evidence for peptidergic co-transmitters (Hökfelt *et al.*, 1980) and for multiple chemical signals in synaptic transmission (Fuxe & Agnati, 1985). It can also explain why the function of the putative endogenous benzodiazepine receptor ligand is impressively enhanced when GABAergic transmission is impaired. Under normal conditions, the primary transmitter GABA might be released in excess. Under such conditions any effect of a system functioning only for fine adjustment might not be very prominent. In conclusion, the hypothesis of the putative benzodiazepine receptor ligand representing a co-transmitter at GABAergic terminals is very plausible and could explain many of the conflicting findings. However, at present few data directly support this hypothesis (Corda *et al.*, 1982; Krespan *et al.*, 1984; Lal & Harris, 1985).

The major remaining controversy centres around the question about the pharmacological properties of the putative endogenous benzodiazepine receptor ligand: is it an agonist or an inverse agonist, or, in other words, is it an endogenous anxiolytic or anxiogenic compound. While points 1 and 2 above strongly favour the presence of an endogenous inverse agonist, points 3 and 5 suggest more the presence of an endogenous antagonist. A final explanation has not yet been given, but three possible hypotheses have been put forward.

In the first hypothesis, Costa's group (Costa *et al.*, 1984) suggested changing the whole system and considering benzodiazepines as antagonists, Ro 15–1788 as a partial agonist, and DBI and several β-carbolines as agonists. This explanation, however, seems fairly unlikely, since it cannot convincingly explain the dualistic and opposite properties of benzodiazepine receptor ligands.

The second hypothesis assumes the presence of only one endogenous ligand but with different pharmacological properties due to the existence of at least two subtypes of benzodiazepine receptors. This hypothesis goes in line with the observation of two biochemically distinct benzodiazepine receptor subtypes with different affinities for some β-carboline derivatives. Beside this difference in affinity, it might be possible that a given benzodiazepine receptor ligand acts at one subtype as an agonist but at the other subtype as an inverse agonist (Sieghart, 1985). This hypothesis might be more likely than the first one. However, different pharmacological properties of the two best characterized benzodiazepine receptor subclasses have not yet been unequivocally demonstrated (Sieghart, 1985).

The last hypothesis is somewhat different and assumes the presence of at least two different endogenous ligands. If we consider that evolution is very economical and does not maintain a biological system unless it is needed, we should ask again why we have this complicated receptor system with the possibility of agonistic and inverse agonistic functions. Why should we not assume that our brain uses both possible pharmacological properties, or why should we not have an endogenous agonist as well as an endogenous inverse agonist, both modulating inhibitory GABAergic neurotransmission in two opposite directions? Evidence for endogenous peptide ligands (but both possibly representing only precursors) functioning as agonist (3000 dalton factor) or as inverse agonist (DBI) has already been presented (§ 6.1.2). Moreover, it has already been demonstrated that the presence of agonistic or inverse agonistic properties can be achieved in the same chemical molecule by only very small structural changes, e.g. for several β-carbolines (Braestrup *et al.*, 1983*a*) or for some pyrazoloquinolines (Yokoyama *et al.*, 1982). In other words, the two different endogenous ligands could be chemically related. Although the concept of two opposing systems (ligands) both existing in a dynamic homeostatic balance, as would be the case with the benzodiazepine receptor system under normal conditions (Davis *et al.*, 1984), is fairly common in nature, the postulated homeostatic balance between two endogenous substances acting at the same receptor system is unusual and, as far as I know, without any other example in biology.

Despite the difficulties mentioned, the last hypothesis seems to be the most attractive, as it explains best the large variety of experimental data regarding the different pharmacological or physiological properties of the putative endogenous ligands of the benzodiazepine receptor. A similar conclusion was reached recently by File & Pellow (1986) in their review of the intrinsic actions of the benzodiazepine receptor antagonist Ro 15–1788, who stated:

> In conclusion, it is possible to account for the unusual pharmacological profile of Ro 15–1788 with a hypothesis of benzodiazepine receptor function requiring the presence of two endogenous ligands with opposing pharmacological effects, both of which can be antagonized by Ro 15–1788; the proportion of these ligands existent at any given time will determine the direction of the effects that Ro 15–1788 will have.

What remains as a final conclusion is the observation that the regulation and control of neuronal function in the CNS seems to be much more complicated than usually described by our concepts of primary inhibitory and excitatory neurotransmitters. If the GABA receptor is functionally modulated for fine adjustment by one or more endogenous benzodiazepine receptor ligands, why should we not postulate a similar system of fine adjustment for other neurotransmitter receptors as well? If this is the case, the benzodiazepine receptor might be one of the first steps in our understanding of a deeper level of regulatory mechanism for chemical neurotransmission beside the classical neurotransmitters and their recognition sites.

9

Future aspects for therapy and research in psychiatry

Many of the future developments and future aspects of benzodiazepine receptor research have already been mentioned in previous chapters. Not all will be reviewed here, since it is the major intention of the present chapter to point specifically in the major directions of future developments rather than to summarize all of them.

9.1 Pharmacotherapy

With the exception of the introduction of more than 20 different benzodiazepines with qualitatively similar but pharmacokinetically different properties, the first 20 years since the introduction of chlordiazepoxid have brought few new aspects in respect to pharmacotherapy with benzodiazepines. This rather negative picture has changed quite significantly during the last few years, since several new benzodiazepine-related drugs have been developed within that time. Some of these have already been introduced into clinical practice.

As might be expected, few new findings have been made regarding *benzodiazepine receptor agonists* like the classical benzodiazepines, since all these compounds are qualitatively fairly similar due to the common receptor mechanism. This might also hold true for some non-benzodiazepine agonists, the drug zopiclone being a typical example. Although having a different chemical structure, this drug comes pharmacologically very close to the classical benzodiazepines, so that effects and side-effects are more similar than different. One has to be very careful that the fact that such drugs are chemically not benzodiazepines is not overestimated when the benefit to risk relationship of these new drugs is compared with that of the classical benzodiazepines.

The future therapeutic use of pure *benzodiazepine receptor antagonists* might be the rapid termination of benzodiazepine overdosing, either accidentally (e.g. suicide) or intentionally (e.g. use of high doses in anaesthesia). The first of these antagonists, the drug Ro 15–1788, will soon be available for clinical application (Haefely, 1985). Whether, beside this rather limited therapeutic potential, benzodiazepine receptor antagonists become useful in the therapy of coma and seizure disorders (see § 6.2.4 and 6.2.5) is very speculative in the present state of our knowledge and experience.

The promising therapeutic potential of the newer *partial benzodiazepine receptor agonists* has already been described in § 3.3. Future research with these substances will show whether their predicted good anxiolytic but low sedative properties can be confirmed. Moreover, carefully controlled studies with these drugs are needed to evaluate the possible lower dependence-producing potential of these compounds relative to the full benzodiazepine receptor agonists.

While the classical benzodiazepines are usually of little benefit in severe depressive disorders (Johnson, 1983; Schatzberg *et al.*, 1983), specific *antidepressive* properties have been claimed for some *triazolo-benzodiazepine derivatives*. A first member of these compounds, alprazolam, has recently been introduced into clinical practice (for a review, see Lader & Davies, 1986). While several controlled clinical studies have shown that alprazolam (for formula, see Fig. 9.1) possesses antidepressive properties, it is presently

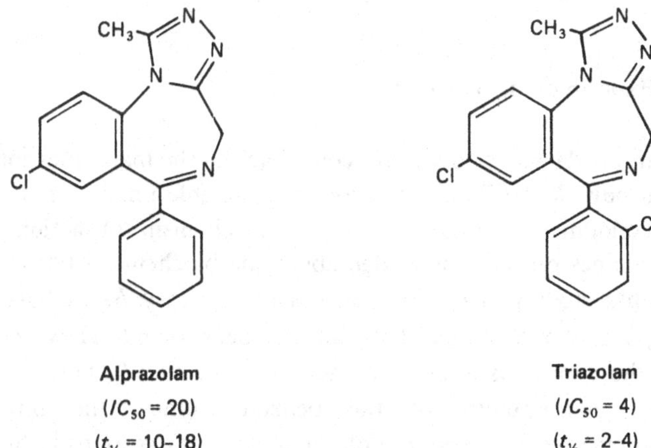

Fig. 9.1. Structural formulae, elimination half-life in man ($t_{1/2}$) and half-maximal inhibitory concentration (in nmol/l) for benzodiazepine receptor binding *in vitro* of the two structurally related triazolo-benzodiazepine derivatives, alprazolam and triazolam.

still a matter of dispute whether these properties distinguish alprazolam from other benzodiazepines, and if they do, to what extent. Moreover, while the possibility of having an anxiolytic benzodiazepine (like alprazolam) with intrinsic antidepressive properties seems to be quite promising with regard to the much less pronounced side-effects of benzodiazepine relative to antidepressive drugs, the benefit to risk relationship is certainly less in favour of alprazolam with regard to withdrawal problems and dependence. Thus, although alprazolam certainly represents a very interesting drug, it still should be used with caution.

To complete this overview, a few CNS active *benzodiazepines which are not benzodiazepines* will also be mentioned. These compounds, although being chemically 1,4-benzodiazepines, do not bind to the benzodiazepine receptor at pharmacologically active concentrations, but affect CNS function via other mechanisms. Examples might be the drug tifluadom, which actually is an opioid (Roemer *et al.*, 1982; Kley *et al.*, 1983), and the thieno-benzodiazepine derivative KC 5944, which is possibly a dopamine receptor antagonist (Ruhland *et al.*, 1985).

In conclusion, as indicated by the data above, a variety of benzodiazepine receptor-related drugs is currently under investigation, which will certainly represent new therapeutic developments when introduced into clinical practice. Moreover, it is important to note that the use of the term 'benzodiazepine' as representative of a chemically and pharmacologically similar group of drugs will not be possible in future.

9.2 Experimental research

In this last section we will come back to the main question asked in the Introduction (Chapter 1) about the possible impact of the recent major developments in respect of the mechanism of action of the benzodiazepines on our knowledge about the biochemical basis of CNS disorders like anxiety, sleep disturbances and epilepsy. As we have learnt, some important new aspects have already been found. However, if we consider the enormous amount of new data we already have about the molecular pharmacology of the benzodiazepines, the impact of benzodiazepine receptor research on the important questions in biological psychiatry research (see above) has been very limited. In my opinion, this is not because there are no relationships between benzodiazepine receptor function and pathological brain function, but because we have only just started to look for such relationships. Possible directions for future research in this area have already been mentioned in many parts of the present book. The few that I regard as most important will be summarized below.

As already outlined in Chapter 6, the major problem with regard to the possible relevance of the benzodiazepine receptor for normal and pathological brain function is the question about the endogenous ligand. Since, today, much evidence suggests the presence of such an endogenous compound, its identification could have an important impact on biological psychiatry research. Pathological changes of the ligand are usually the more likely mechanism than changes of its receptor.

On the other hand, pathological changes of the receptor itself are certainly possible, as indicated by a variety of data from animals and *post mortem* samples of human brain. In many of these studies, the pathological changes seemed to be a specific response of the benzodiazepine receptor only and were not accompanied by similar changes of the GABA receptor. However, the interpretations were sometimes difficult, since not all the studies determined the low-affinity GABA receptors as the sites relevant for benzodiazepine receptor function. Since the benzodiazepine–GABA–barbiturate receptor complex has recently been solubilized and purified with well-preserved interactions between the three recognition sites (Schoch *et al.*, 1984; Sigel *et al.*, 1984), the development of specific antibodies against each of the three recognition sites of this multifunctional complex has become possible. Using such specific antibodies and immunohistological techniques, it will become possible in the near future to evaluate to what extent all three recognition sites of this postsynaptic part of GABAergic synapses are regulated independently from one another.

Since these techniques will be limited to animal studies or studies using *post mortem* brain samples, another important aspect for future studies will be the receptor visualization using positron emission tomography techniques, especially if the spatial resolution of this method can be increased and if other ligands, especially to visualize the GABA receptor, become available. Despite their limited spatial resolution, this method has the major advantage that changes and especially acute changes of benzodiazepine receptor properties can be investigated in the patient. The latter point seems to me of special importance since several of the animal data suggest changes of the benzodiazepine receptor as a response to different pathological stimuli. Moreover, interesting data about acute changes of low-affinity GABA receptors by a putative endogenous benzodiazepine receptor ligand as a specific response to stress have also been reported (see § 7.2.3). It seems likely that such acute adaptive changes of receptor properties represent an important aspect of normal brain function, and thus might be altered in the course of CNS disorders. As judged from the animal data, these adaptive changes are quite pronounced. Thus, if present in human brain also, such changes should be detectable with the PET techniques available, despite their limited sensitivity.

In conclusion, promising aspects exist for future research in biological psychiatry. Returning to Emil Kraepelin (1892), we have already learned much 'about the specific effect of a given drug on a specific psychic symptom'. There is a good chance that this knowledge will finally lead us to understand the 'true nature of this symptom' within the next few years.

APPENDIX 1

The benzodiazepine radioreceptor assay: a rapid and sensitive method to detect benzodiazepines in biological tissues

As described in § 2.1, there is usually a very good correlation between the concentration of a given benzodiazepine derivative and the inhibition of specific radioligand binding to the benzodiazepine receptor. Moreover, if the experimental conditions (tissue, buffer, pH, temperature, etc.) are well standardized, the same ligand concentration will give about the same inhibition of specific radioligand binding from experiment to experiment and from day to day. It is obvious that such a stable effect can be used to assay an unknown concentration of a benzodiazepine derivative. Such assays, which represent something between a bioassay and a radioimmunoassay, are called radioreceptor assays, and have been described for drugs like neuroleptics, β-blockers and anticholinergics (Perret & Simon, 1984). Moreover, several authors have reported radioreceptor assays for the determination of benzodiazepines in human plasma or CSF (Hunt *et al.*, 1979; Owen *et al.*, 1979; Jochemsen *et al.*, 1983; Lascelles, 1983; Tyma *et al.*, 1984).

There are two general applications for such a benzodiazepine radioreceptor assay. First, if the benzodiazepine derivative is known and is not metabolized to active derivatives, the radioreceptor assay can be used to quantify the plasma concentration of this derivative by the use of a standard curve with the same derivative. Second, in most cases, present in plasma is not only the parent benzodiazepine derivative but also one or more active metabolites. Moreover, in many cases of benzodiazepine poisoning, more than one benzodiazepine has been taken. In such cases, all active compounds will inhibit benzodiazepine receptor binding and thus will be 'seen' by the radioreceptor assay. Results cannot be expressed as concentration of a given compound, but are usually expressed as equivalents with respect to a standard compound. Since the receptor 'sees' the drugs in relation to their affinity and since the affinity correlates very well with their therapeutic activity, the radioreceptor gives a very good estimate of the therapeutically or toxicologically relevant level of benzodiazepine activity in human plasma.

It is a major advantage that the receptor 'sees' the benzodiazepines in relation to their therapeutic activity. This is not the case for radioimmunoassays of benzodiazepines, which also 'see' more than one benzodiazepine derivative, but immunoreactivity usually does not correlate with therapeutic activity (Jacqmin & Lesne, 1984; de Blas *et al.*, 1985). In conclusion, the benzodiazepine radioreceptor assay measures all therapeutically active benzodiazepine derivatives and their active metabolites present in human plasma in relation to their therapeutic activity, and thus gives an excellent estimate of the overall benzodiazepine activity in plasma.

A1.1 Methodological aspects

The major advantage of the benzodiazepine radioreceptor assay is its simplicity. It can easily be learned in a relatively short time. The only apparatus needed is a liquid scintillation counter, which is available today in most laboratories. If bovine brain tissue is used as described below, no facilities to keep experimental animals are needed. The specific method is as follows.

Tissue preparation

Fresh bovine brains can easily be obtained from local slaughterhouses. The cortex (frontal, temporal and occipital) is dissected on ice and stored in 1 g aliquots at –20 °C. Under these conditions, the tissue is stable for at least 3 months. For the binding assay, 1 g aliquots of the bovine cortex tissue are homogenized in about 50 ml 50 nmol/l Tris-HCl buffer at pH 7.4. After centrifugation at 48 000 × *g* for about 10 min., the supernatant is discarded and the pellet resuspended in about 150 ml 50 mmol/l Tris-HCl buffer pH 7.4. The tissue homogenate can be stored on ice (4 °C) for 1 or 2 h.

Binding assay

For the binding assay, 900 μl of the tissue homogenate are incubated for 60 min. at 4 °C with 50 μl [^{3}H]FNT (to give a final concentration of about

0.3 nmol/l) and either 50 μl buffer (total binding), or 50 μl cold diazepam (to give a final concentration of 10 μmol/l as blank to determine non-specific binding, see Fig. 2.2), or 50 μl of the dried ethyl acetate extract of plasma in buffer (experimental values), or 50 μl buffer containing cold diazepam (to give final diazepam concentrations ranging from 3 to 30 nmol/l as standard curve, see Fig. A1.1). The incubation is terminated by rapid

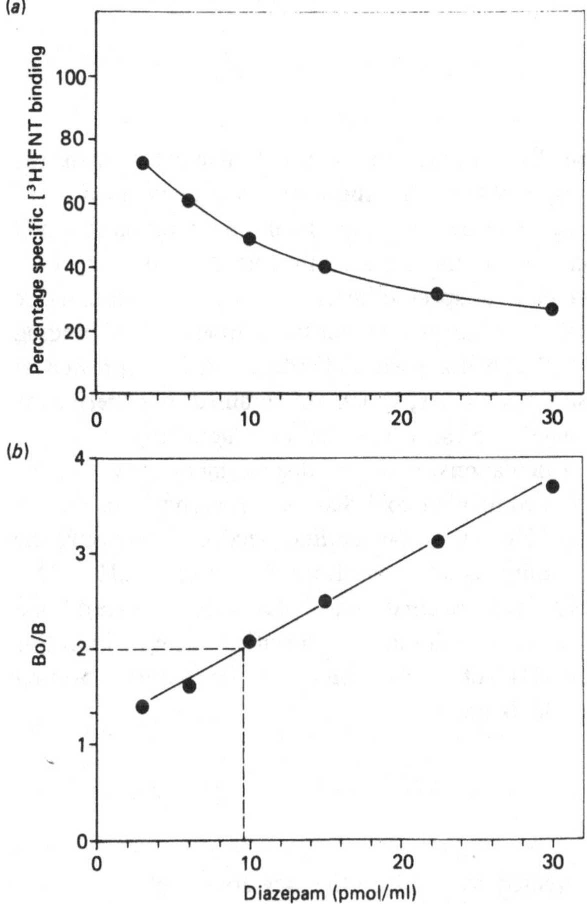

Fig. A1.1. The effect of increasing concentrations of diazepam on specific [^{3}H]FNT binding to bovine cortex homogenates. Application for a radioreceptor assay. (*a*) Linear plot. (*b*) Plot of the diazepam concentration (pmol/ml, abscissa) versus the quotient between the amount of specific binding in the absence and the presence of diazepam (Bo/B, ordinate) which results in a straight line for the diazepam concentration range indicated. This plot can be used to express benzodiazepine-like activity in human plasma in diazepam equivalents, if human plasma extracts are diluted to inhibit specific binding of the radioligand within the linear range.

filtration through Whatman GF-B filters under slight vacuum. The filters are washed three times with 3 ml of the ice-cold incubation buffer, placed in minivials, and dried for 30 min. at 60 °C. Radioactivity on the filters is extracted into 4 ml of a Triton-containing scintillation fluid by standing overnight. Under these conditions, counting efficiency is similar for each sample and the measured counts (CPMs) can be used directly for calculation.

Calculations

The level of non-specific binding (binding not associated with the benzodiazepine receptor) is obtained for the assay system described above by the probes containing the blank (diazepam, final concentration 10 μmol/l). The CPMs for non-specific binding are substracted from each probe to obtain the respective data for specific (receptor-associated) binding (see Fig. 2.2). Taking specific binding obtained for the samples of total binding by this way as 100%, all data for specific binding can be expressed as percentages of these standard values, which are obtained by experiments where no displacing ligand is present (see total binding in Fig. 2.1).

Using these simple calculations, a typical displacement curve will be obtained for the samples containing cold diazepam ranging from 3 to 30 nmol/l (see Fig. A1.1*a*). This curve can be linearized by expressing the amount of specific binding as quotient Bo/B (see Fig. A1.1*b*). This relationship now serves as standard curve and all plasma extracts are diluted (if necessary) to give values for inhibition of specific binding within this linear range (Fig. A1.1*b*). Data of an unknown plasma sample are expressed in diazepam pico-equivalents per ml.

Plasma extraction

1 ml of plasma is extracted with 2 ml ethyl acetate. 1 ml of the ethyl acetate extract is evaporated to dryness. The residue is dissolved in 0.5 ml Tris-HCl buffer pH 7.4. If 50 μl of this extract are used for the binding assay, the final concentration of the benzodiazepine extracted from plasma in the assay system will be one-twentieth of its concentration in the plasma. In many cases, this will be sufficient. If a higher sensitivity is desired, the binding assay can be made directly in a glass tube where 1 ml of the ethyl acetate extract has been evaporated to dryness. In this case, the

concentration in the assay system will be only half of the original plasma concentration. Using this system, all benzodiazepines which we have checked are extracted completely (see Table 2.1).

Sensitivity

The sensitivity of the assay system described above is usually high enough to detect therapeutic plasma levels. The sensitivity can easily be increased if more plasma is extracted, but this will rarely be needed. If the assay is performed in the same tube where 1 ml of ethyl acetate extract has been evaporated, benzodiazepine plasma levels equivalent to 10 ng/ml of diazepam can easily be determined (see Table A1.1).

Table A1.1 *Diazepam equivalents of benzodiazepine plasma levels as determined by radioreceptor assay*

Inhibitory concentrations 50% (IC_{50}) of several benzodiazepines as inhibitors of specific [^{3}H]FNT binding to bovine cortex homogenates and the calculated plasma concentration equivalents to diazepam (10 ng/ml) of several benzodiazepines, when determined using the same system as radioreceptor assay.

Benzodiazepine	IC_{50} (nmol/l)	Plasma level equivalent to diazepam 10 ng/ml (ng/ml)
Alprazolam	8	9
Bromazepam	30	33
Clobazam	310	320
Clonazepam	3	3
Diazepam	10	10
Desmethyldiazepam	20	19
Flunitrazepam	3	3
Nitrazepam	30	29
Lorazepam	3	3
Ro 15–1788	1	1
Temazepam	40	41
Tetrazepam	70	69
Triazolam	4	5

Practicability

In our experience, the radioreceptor assay is a very simple method to obtain a reliable value about the benzodiazepine-like activity present in plasma or any other biological tissue. Since other drugs will not bind to the benzodiazepine receptor in the usual therapeutic concentration range, this method is highly specific for benzodiazepines and related compounds. However, in terms of analytical accuracy, classical methods like gas or liquid chromatography might be superior. Thus, if a specific benzodiazepine drug should be analysed in plasma with high accuracy, these classical methods might be more suitable. On the other hand, if the clinician wants to know very quickly how much benzodiazepine is present in a given blood sample, and where it does not matter which specific benzodiazepine derivative is present, the radioreceptor assay is the method of choice.

A1.2 Some practical implications and uses

As already mentioned, the major advantage of the benzodiazepine radioreceptor assay is that it sees all benzodiazepines and their active metabolites present in plasma in relation to their clinical activity. Thus, it is less suitable to study classical plasma concentration versus time kinetics, since not only one but all active compounds are determined. On the other hand, it seems the method of choice if plasma concentration versus effect kinetics are to be determined, since the effect is the final result of all active compounds (parent drug and metabolites) in plasma. The latter point seems to be of special importance, since up to now most attempts to correlate plasma levels of benzodiazepines with pharmacodynamic effects in man, or even with therapeutic response, have not been very successful (for a review, see Klotz, 1984). Although it is quite clear that a large variety of different factors contributes to these poor correlations, some recent and preliminary data suggest that at least one area of these problems might be overcome if the radioreceptor assay is used instead of one of the classical analytical methods measuring the parent compound and possibly one (usually the main) metabolite (Aranko *et al.*, 1984; Saletu *et al.*, 1984).

While the use of the benzodiazepine radioreceptor assay to determine possible relationships between plasma levels and pharmacodynamic effects is certainly more of scientific than of practical interest, there are some clinical situations where an exact knowledge about the plasma concentration of benzodiazepines is desirable. These situations are certainly the exception, as there is usually no need for therapeutic drug monitoring in the case of benzodiazepines (Lascelles, 1983). One such situation is overdosage with benzodiazepines, where a fast knowledge about the active plasma level might be helpful (Aaaltonen & Scheinin, 1982). Another situation might be 'negative' compliance in cases of benzodiazepine dependence and especially during gradual withdrawal in cases of benzodiazepine dependence, which is usually done under the control of the plasma levels (Tyrer *et al.*, 1983; Ashton, 1984; Winokur & Rickels, 1984). In both of these cases, the radioreceptor assay might represent a valuable tool to determine whether more than the prescribed number of tablets has been taken. In conclusion, in all cases when it is important to know how much benzodiazepine activity rather than what specific plasma concentration of a given benzodiazepine are present, the benzodiazepine radioreceptor assay represents an interesting alternative to classical analytical methods.

APPENDIX 2

Abbreviations

B_{max} maximal binding capacity of a receptor ligand in a given tissue preparation, synonymous with receptor density.

BZ_1 benzodiazepine receptor subclass with high densities in the cerebellum of many species.

BZ_2 benzodiazepine receptor subclass with high densities in the hippocampus of many species.

Cl 218 872 3-methyl-3-(trifluoromethyl)phenyl -1,2,3-triazolo 4,3-b pyridazine, a benzodiazepine receptor agonist with some selectivity for the BZ_1 subclass.

CNS central nervous system.

DBI diazepam binding inhibitor, a putative endogenous ligand of the benzodiazepine receptor.

[^{3}H]diaz tritiated diazepam, a radioligand for the benzodiazepine receptor.

DMCM methyl-6,7-dimethoxy-β-carboline-3-carboxylate, an inverse benzodiazepine receptor agonist.

β-ECC ethyl β-carboline-3-carboxylate, an inverse benzodiazepine receptor agonist.

ED_{50} effective dose 50%, pharmacological dose which gives the desired effect in 50% of the experiments.

FG 7142 *N*-methyl-β-carboline-3-carboxamide, an inverse benzodiazepine receptor agonist.

[^{3}H]FNT tritiated flunitrazepam, a radioligand for the benzodiazepine receptor.

GABA γ-aminobutyric acid, an inhibitory neurotransmitter.

5-HT 5-hydroxytryptamine, serotonin, a neurotransmitter.

IC_{50} inhibitory concentration 50% pharmacological concentration which gives 50% of a given maximal effect.

IPSP inhibitory postsynaptic potential.

K_D dissociation constant.

K_i inhibition constant.

β-MCC methyl β-carboline-3-carboxylate, an inverse agonist of the benzodiazepine receptor.

PK 11195 1-(2-chlorophenyl)-N-methyl-(1-methyl propyl)-3 isoquinolinecarboxamide, a putative antagonist of peripheral benzodiazepine binding sites.

β-PrCC propyl β-carboline-3-carboxylate, a benzodiazepine receptor antagonist.

Ro 5–4864 4′-chlorodiazepam, a putative agonist of peripheral benzodiazepine binding sites.

Ro 15–1788 ethyl 8-fluoro-5,6-dihydro-5-methyl-6-oxo-4H-imidazo (1,5-a)-1,4-benzodiazepine-3-carboxylate, a benzodiazepine receptor antagonist.

$t_{1/2}$ elimination half-life.

ZK 93 426 ethyl 5-isopropoxy-4-methyl-β-carboline-3-carboxylate, a benzodiazepine receptor antagonist.

REFERENCES

Aaltonen, L., Erkkola, R. & Kanto, J. (1983). Benzodiazepine receptors in the human fetus. *Biology of the Neonate*, **44**, 54–7.

Aaltonen, L. & Scheinin, M. (1982). Application of radioreceptor assay of benzodiazepines for toxicology. *Acta Pharmacologica et Toxicologica*, **50**, 206–12.

Abbracchio, M.P., Balduini, W., Coen, E., Lombardelli, G., Peruzzi, I. & Cattabeni, F. (1983). Chronic chlordiazepoxide treatment on adult and newborn rats: effect on the GABA–benzodiazepine receptor complex. In *Benzodiazepine recognition site ligands: biochemistry and pharmacology*, ed. G. Biggio & E. Costa, pp. 227–37. New York: Raven Press.

Airaksinen, M.M. & Kari, I. (1981). β-carbolines, psycho-active compounds in the mammalian body. Part 1: Occurrence, origin and metabolism. Part 2: Effects. *Medical Biology*, **59**, 21–34 and 190–211.

Airaksinen, M.M., & Mikkonen, E. (1980). Affinity of β-carbolines on rat brain benzodiazepine and opiate binding sites. *Medical Biology*, **58**, 341–4.

Akil, H., Watson, St J., Young, E., Lewis, M.E., Khachaturian, H. & Walker, J.M. (1984). Endogenous opioids: biology and function. *Annual Reviews of Neuroscience*, **7**, 223–55.

Alho, H., Costa, E., Ferrero, P., Fujimoto, M., Cosenza-Murphy, D. & Guiditto, A. (1985). Diazepam-binding inhibitor: a neuropeptide located in selected neuronal populations of rat brain. *Science*, **229**, 178–82.

Ally, A.I., Manku, M.S., Horrobin, D.D., Karmali, R.A., Morgan, R.O. & Karmazyn, M. (1977). Thromboxane A_2 as a possible natural ligand for benzodiazepine receptors. *Neuroscience Letters*, **7**, 31–4.

Aranko, K., Mattila, M.J., Sepplälä, T. & Aranko, S. (1984). The contribution of the active metabolites to the tolerance developing to diazepam in man: relationship to bioassayed serum benzodiazepine levels. *Medical Biology*, **62**, 277–84.

Armando, I., Barontini, M., Levin, G., Simsolo, R., Glover, V. & Sandler, M. (1984). Exercise increases endogenous urinary monoamine oxidase benzodiazepine receptor ligand inhibitory activity in normal children. *Journal of the Autonomic Nervous System*, **11**, 95–100.

Asano, T. & Mizutani, A. (1980). Brain benzodiazepine receptors and their rapid changes after seizures in the mongolian gerbil. *Japanese Journal of Pharmacology*, **30**, 783–8.

Asano, T. & Ogasawara, N. (1982). Prostaglandins as possible endogenous ligands of benzodiazepine receptor. *European Journal of Pharmacology*, **80**, 271–4.

Asano, T. & Spector, S. (1979). Identification of inosine and hypoxanthine as endogenous ligands for the brain benzodiazepine-binding sites. *Proceedings of the National Academy of Sciences, USA*, **76**, 977–81.

Ashton, H. (1984). Benzodiazepine withdrawal: an unfinished story. *British Medical Journal*, **288**, 1135–40.

Atterwill, C.K. & Nutt, D.J. (1983). Thyroid hormones do not alter rat brain benzodiazepine receptor function *in vivo*. *Journal of Pharmacy and Pharmacology*, **35**, 767–8.

Bansky, G., Meier, P.J., Ziegler, W.H., Walser, H., Schmid, M. & Huber, M. (1985). Reversal of hepatic coma by benzodiazepine antagonist (Ro 15–1788). *The Lancet* **i**, 1324–5.

Baraldi, M. & Zeneroli, M.L. (1982). Experimental encephalopathy: changes in GABA. *Science*, **216**, 427–31.

Baraldi, M., Zeneroli, M.L., Ventura, E., Penne, A., Pinelli, G., Ricci, P. & Santi, M. (1984). Supersensitivity of benzodiazepine receptors in hepatic encephalopathy due to fulminant hepatic failure in the rat: reversal by a benzodiazepine antagonist. *Clinical Science*, **67**, 167–75.

Barbaccia, M.L., Gandolfi, O., Chuang, D.M. & Costa, E. (1983). Modulation of neuronal serotonin uptake by a putative endogenous ligand of imipramine recognition sites. *Proceedings of the National Academy of Sciences, USA*, **80**, 5134–8.

Barker, J.L., Gratz, E., Owen, D.G. & Study, R.E. (1984). Pharmacological effects of clinically important drugs on the excitability of cultured mouse spinal neurons. In *Actions and interactions of GABA and benzodiazepines*, ed. N.G. Bowery, pp. 203–16. New York: Raven Press.

Barr, G.A. & Lithgow, T. (1983). Effect of age on benzodiazepine-induced behavioural convulsions in rats. *Nature*, **5907**, 431–2.

Baumeister, A.A. & Frye, G.D. (1984). The biochemical basis of the behavioural disorder in the Lesch-Nyhan syndrome. *Neuroscience and Behavioral Reviews*, **9**, 169–78.

Beaumont, K., Cheung, A.K., Geller, M.L. & Fanestil, D.D. (1983). Inhibitors of peripheral-type benzodiazepine receptors present in human urine and plasma ultrafiltrates. *Life Sciences*, **33**, 1375–84.

Bellantuono, C., Reggi, V., Tognoni, G. & Garattini, S. (1980). Benzodiazepines: clinical pharmacology and therapeutic use. *Drugs*, **19**, 195–219.

Bénavidès, J., Guilloux, F., Allam, D.E., Uzan, A., Mizoule, J., Renault, C., Dubroeucq, M.C., Gueremy, C. & Le Fur, G. (1984*a*). Opposite effects of an agonist, Ro 15–4864, and an antagonist, PK 11195, of the peripheral type benzodiazepine binding sites on audiogenic seizures in *DBA/2J* mice. *Life Sciences*, **34**, 2613–20.

Bénavidès, J., Quarteronet, D., Plouin, P.-F., Imbault, F., Phan, T., Uzan, A., Renault, C., Dubroeuco, M. C., Gueremy, C., Le Fur, G. (1984*b*). Characterization of peripheral type benzodiazepine binding sites in human and rat platelets by using [^{3}H]PK 11195. Studies in hypertensive patients. *Biochemical Pharmacology*, **33**, 2467–72.

Bennett, J.P., Jr., Enna, S.J., Bylund, D.B., Gillin, J.C., Wyatt, R.J. & Snyder, S.H. (1979). Neurotransmitter receptors in frontal cortex of schizophrenics. *Archives of General Psychiatry*, **36**, 927–34.

Biggio, G., Corda, M.G., Concas, A. & Gessa, G.L. (1981*a*). Denervation supersensitivity for benzodiazepine receptors in the rat substantia nigra. *Brain Research*, **220**, 344–9.

Biggio, G., Corda, M.G., Lamberti, C. & Gessa, G.L. (1979). Changes in benzodiazepine receptors following GABAergic denervation of substantia nigra. *European Journal of Pharmacology*, **58**, 215–16.

Biggio, G., Concas, A., Serra, M., Salis, M., Corda, M.G., Nurchi, V., Crisponi, C. & Gessa, G.L. (1984). Stress and β-carbolines decrease the density of low affinity GABA binding sites; an effect reversed by diazepam. *Brain Research*, **305**, 13–18.

Biggio, G., Guarneri, P. & Corda, M.G. (1981*b*). Benzodiazepine and GABA receptors in the retina: effect of light and dark adaptation. *Brain Research*, **216**, 210–14.

Biscoe, T.J. & Fry, J.P. (1984). GABA and benzodiazepine receptors in neurologically mutant mice. In *Actions and interactions of GABA and benzodiazepines*, ed. N.G. Bowery, pp. 217–37. New York: Raven Press.

Biscoe, T.J., Fry, J.P. & Rickets, C. (1984). Changes in benzodiazepine receptor binding as seen autoradiographically in the central nervous system of the spastic mouse. *Journal of Physiology*, **352**, 509–16.

Blaha, L. & Brückmann, J.U. (1983). Benzodiazepines in the treatment of anxiety (*Angst*): European experiences. In *The benzodiazepines, from molecular biology to clinical practice*, ed. E. Costa, pp. 311–23. New York: Raven Press.

Blaschke, G., Kley, H. & Müller, W.E. (1986). Optical resolution of the benzodiazepines camazepam and ketazolam and receptor affinity of the enantiomers. *Arzneimittel-Forschung*, **36**, 893–4.

Boast, C.A., Bernard, P.S., Barbaz, B.S. & Bergen, K.M. (1983). The neuropharmacology of various diazepam antagonists. *Neuropharmacology*, **128**, 1511–21.

Bold, J.M., Gardner, C.R. & Walker, R.J. (1985). Central effects of nicotinamide and inosine which are not mediated through benzodiazepine receptors. *British Journal of Pharmacology*, **84**, 689–96.

Bolger, G.T., Weissman, B.A., Lueddens, H., Basile, A.S., Mantione, C.R., Barrett, J.E., Witkin, J.M., Paul, St M. & Skolnick, P. (1985). Late evolutionary appearance of peripheral-type binding sites for benzodiazepines. *Brain Research*, **338**, 366–70.

Borbe, H.O., Fehske, K.J., Müller, W.E., Nover, A. & Wollert, U. (1982). The demonstration of several neurotransmitter and drug receptors in human retina. *Comparative Biochemistry and Physiology*, **1**, 117–19.

Borbe, H.O., Müller, W.E. & Wollert, U. (1980). The identification of benzodiazepine receptors with brain-like specificity in bovine retina. *Brain Research*, **182**, 466–9.

Bormann, J. & Clapham, D.E. (1985). γ-Aminobutyric acid receptor channels in adrenal chromaffin cells: a patch-clamp study. *Proceedings of the National Academy of Sciences, USA*, **82**, 2168–72.

Bossmann, H.B., Penney, D.P., Case, K.R., Distefano, P., Averill, K. (1978). Diazepam receptor specific binding of [^{3}H]diazepam and [^{3}H]flunitrazepam to rat brain subfractions. *FEBS Letters*, **87**, 199–202.

Bowdler, J.M. & Green, A.R. (1982). Regional rat brain benzodiazepine receptor number and γ-aminobutyric acid concentration following a convulsion. *British Journal of Pharmacology*, **76**, 291–8.

Bowery, N.G., Hill, D.R., Hudson, A.L., Price, G.W., Turnbull, M.J. & Wilkin, G.P. (1984). Heterogeneity of mammalian GABA receptors. In *Actions and interactions of GABA and benzodiazepines*, ed. N.G. Bowery, pp. 81–108. New York: Raven Press.

Bowling, A.C. & DeLorenzo, R.J. (1982). Micromolar affinity benzodiazepine receptors: identification and characterization in central nervous system. *Science*, **216**, 1247–50.

Braestrup, C., Albrechtsen, R. & Squires, R.F., (1977). High densities of benzodiazepine receptors in human cortical areas, *Nature*, **5639**, 702–4.

Braestrup, C. & Nielsen, M. (1978). Ontogenetic development of benzodiazepine receptors in the rat brain. *Brain Research*, **147**, 170–3.

Braestrup, C. & Nielsen, M. (1981). GABA reduces binding of ^{3}H-methyl β-carboline-3-carboxylate to brain benzodiazepine receptors. *Nature*, **294**, 472–4.

Braestrup, C. & Nielsen, M. (1983). Benzodiazepine receptors. In *Handbook of psychopharmacology, Vol. 17*, ed. L.L. Iversen, S.D. Inversen & S.H. Snyder, pp. 285–384. New York: Plenum Press.

Braestrup, C., Nielsen, M., Honoré, T., Jensen, L.H. & Petersen, E.N. (1983*a*). Benzodiazepine receptor ligand with positive and negative efficacy. *Neuropharmacology*, **22**, 1451–7.

Braestrup, C., Nielsen, M., Nielsen, E.B. & Lyon, M. (1979). Benzodiazepine receptors in the brain as affected by different experimental stresses: the changes are small and not unidirectional. *Psychopharmacology*, **65**, 273–7.

Braestrup, C., Nielsen, M. & Olsen, C.E. (1980). Urinary and brain β-carboline-3-carboxylates as potent inhibitors of brain benzodiazepine receptors. *Proceedings of the National Academy of Sciences, USA*, **77**, 2288–92.

Braestrup, C., Nielsen, M. & Squires, R.F. (1978). No changes in rat benzodiazepine receptors after withdrawal from continuous treatment with lorazepam and diazepam. *Life Sciences*, **24**, 347–50.

Braestrup, C., Schmiechen, R., Neef, G., Nielsen, M. & Petersen, E.N. (1982). Interaction of convulsive ligands with benzodiazepine receptors. *Science*, **216**, 1241–3.

Braestrup, C., Schmiechen, R., Nielsen, M. & Petersen, E.N. (1983*b*). Benzodiazepine receptor ligands, receptor occupancy, pharmacological effect and GABA receptor coupling. In *Pharmacology of benzodiazepines*, ed. E. Usdin, P. Skolnik, J.F. Tallman, D. Greenblatt & S. Paul, pp. 71–85. Weinheim: Verlag Chemie.

Braestrup, C. & Squires, R.F. (1977). Specific benzodiazepine receptors in rat brain characterized by high-affinity [^{3}H]diazepam binding, *Proceedings of the National Academy of Sciences, USA*, **74**, 3805–9.

Braestrup, C. & Squires, R.F. (1978). Pharmacological characterization of benzodiazepine receptors in the brain. *European Journal of Pharmacology*, **48**, 263–70.

Braunwald, E. (1982). Mechanism of action of calcium-channel-blocking agents. *The New England Journal of Medicine*, **307**, 1618–27.

Burnham, W.M., Niznik, H.B., Okazaki, M.M. & Kish, S.J. (1983). Binding of ^{3}H-flunitrazepam and ^{3}H-Ro 5–4864 to crude homogenates of amygdala-kindled rat brain: two months post-seizures. *Brain Research*, **279**, 359–62.

Carlen, P.L., Gurevich, N. & Polc, P. (1983). The excitatory effects of the specific benzodiazepine antagonist Ro 14–7347 measured intracellularly in hippocampal CA1 cells. *Brain Research*, **271**, 115–19.

Carlsson, A. (1978). Antipsychotic drugs, neurotransmitters, and schizophrenia. *American Journal of Psychiatry*, **135**, 164–72.

Catalan, J. & Gath, D.H. (1985). Benzodiazepines in general practice: time for a decision. *British Medical Journal*, **290**, 1374–6.

Chan, C.Y. & Farb, D.H. (1985). Modulation of neurotransmitter action: control of the γ-aminobutyric acid response through the benzodiazepine receptor. *The Journal of Neuroscience*, **5**, 2365–73.

Chang, R.L., Tran, V.T. & Snyder, S.H. (1980). Neurotransmitter receptor localizations: brain lesion induced alterations in benzodiazepine, GABA, β-adrenergic and histamine H_1-receptor binding. *Brain Research*, **190**, 95–110.

Cheetham, S.C., Crompton, M.R., Katopa, C.L.E., Horton, R.W. & Reynolds, G.P. (1985). $GABA_A$ and benzodiazepine binding sites in the cortex of depressed suicide victims. *British Journal of Pharmacology*, **86**, 593 P.

Chiu, P., Chiu, S. & Mishra, R.K. (1984). Characteristics of [^{3}H]propyl β-carboline-3-carboxylate binding to benzodiazepine receptors in human brain. *Research Communications in Chemical Pathology and Pharmacology*, **44**, 199–213.

Chiu, T.H. & Rosenberg, H.C. (1978). Reduced diazepam binding following chronic benzodiazepine treatment. *Life Sciences*, **23**, 1153–8.

Colello, G.D., Hockenbery, D.M., Bosmann, H.B., Fuchs, S. & Folkers, K. (1978). Competitive inhibition of benzodiazepine binding by fractions from porcine brain, *Proceedings of the National Academy of Sciences, USA*, **75**, 6319–23.

Comar, D., Maziere, M., Godot, J.M., Berger, C.G., Soussaline, F., Menini, C., Arfel, G. & Naquet, R. (1979). Visualisation of ^{11}C-flunitrazepam displacement in the brain of the live baboon. *Nature*, **280**, 329–31.

Concas, A., Salis, M. & Biggio, G. (1983). Brain benzodiazepine receptors increase after chronic ethyl-β-carboline-3-carboxylate. *Life Sciences*, **32**, 1175–82.

Concas, A., Corda, M.G. & Biggio, G. (1985*a*). Involvement of benzodiazepine recognition sites in the foot shock-induced decrease of low-affinity GABA receptors in the rat cerebral cortex. *Brain Research*, **341**, 50–6.

Concas, A., Serra, M., Crisponi, G., Nurchi, V., Corda, M.G. & Biggio, G. (1985*b*). Changes in the characteristics of low-affinity GABA binding sites elicited by Ro 15–1788. *Life Sciences*, **36**, 329–37.

Conti-Tronconi, B.M. & Raftery, M.A. (1982). The nicotinic cholinergic receptor: correlation of molecular structure with functional properties. *Annual Reviews of Biochemistry*, **51**, 491–530.

Corda, M.G., Costa, E. & Guidotti, A. (1982). Specific proconvulsant action of an imidazobenzodiazepine (Ro 15–1788) on isoniazid convulsions. *Neuropharmacology*, **21**, 91–4.

Corda, M.G., Ferrari, M., Guidotti, A., Konkel, D. & Costa, E. (1984). Isolation, purification and partial sequence of a neuropeptide (diazepam-binding inhibitor) precursor of an anxiogenic putative ligand for benzodiazepine recognition site. *Neuroscience Letters*, **47**, 319–24.

Costa, E. (1983). Concluding remarks: are benzodiazepine recognition sites functional entities for the action of endogenous effectors or merely drug receptors? In *Benzodiazepine recognition site ligands: biochemistry and pharmacology*, ed. G. Biggio & E. Costa, pp. 249–53. New York: Raven Press.

Costa, E., Corda, M.G. & Guidotti, A. (1983). On a brain polypeptide functioning as a putative effector for the recognition sites of benzodiazepine and β-carboline derivatives. *Neuropharmacology*, **22**, 1481–92.

Costa, E., Ferrari, M., Ferrero, P. & Guidotti, A. (1984). Multiple signals in GABAergic transmission: pharmacological consequences. *Neuropharmacology*, **23**, 989–91.

Costa, E., Guidotti, A. & Mao, C.C. (1975). Evidence for involvement of GABA in the action of benzodiazepines: studies on rat cerebellum. In *Mechanism of action of benzodiazepines*, ed. E. Costa & P. Greengard, pp. 113–30. New York: Raven Press.

Coupet, J., Rauh, C.E., Lippa, A.S. & Beer, B. (1981). The effects of acute administration of diazepam on the binding of [^{3}H]diazepam and [^{3}H]GABA to rat cortical membranes. *Pharmacology, Biochemistry & Behavior*, **15**, 965–8.

Coyle, J.T. & Schwarz, R. (1976). Lesions of striatal neurones with kainic acid provide a model for Huntington's chorea. *Nature*, **263**, 244–6.

Crawley, J.N. (1983). Animal behavioral analysis of putative endogenous ligands. In *Pharmacology of benzodiazepines*, ed. E. Usdin, P. Skolnick, J.F. Tallman, D. Greenblatt & S. Paul, pp. 549–59. Weinheim: Verlag Chemie.

Crawley, J.N. & Davis, L.G. (1982). Baseline exploratory activity predicts anxiolytic responsiveness to diazepam in five mouse strains. *Brain Research Bulletin*, **8**, 609–12.

Crawley, J.N., Marangos, P.J., Stivers, J. & Goodwin, F.K. (1982). Chronic clonazepam administration induces benzodiazepine receptor subsensitivity. *Neuropharmacology*, **21**, 85–9.

Crow, T.J. (1982) Schizophrenia. In *Disorders of neurohumoral transmission*, ed. by T.J. Crow, pp. 287–340. London: Academic Press.

Crow, T.J., Cross, A.J., Cooper, S.J., Deakin, J.F.W., Ferrier, I.N., Johnson, J.A., Joseph, M.H., Owen, F.M., Poulter, M., Lothouse, R., Corsellis, J.A.N., Chambers, D.R., Blessed, G., Perry, E.K., Perry, R.H. & Tomlinson, B.E. (1984). Neurotransmitter receptors and monoamine metabolites in the brains of patients with Alzheimer-type dementia and depression and suicides. *Neuropharmacology*, **23**, 1561–9.

Cumin, R., Bonetti, E.P., Scherschlicht, R. & Haefely, W.E. (1982). Use of the specific benzodiazepine antagonist Ro 15–1788 in studies of physiological dependence on benzodiazepines. *Experientia*, **38**, 833–4.

Damm, H.W., Müller, W.E. & Wollert, U. (1979). Is the benzodiazepine receptor purinergic? *European Journal of Pharmacology*, **55**, 331–3.

Darragh, A., Lambe, R., O'Boyle, C., Kenny, M. & Brick. I. (1983). Absence of central effects in man of benzodiazepine antagonist Ro 15–1788. *Psychopharmacology*, **80**, 192–5.

Davis, A. (1984). Molecular aspects of the imipramine 'receptor'. *Experientia*, **40**, 782–94.

Davis, L.G. (1983). Is a peptide the natural ligand for the benzodiazepine receptor? In *Pharmacology of benzodiazepines*, ed. E. Usdin, P. Skolnick, J.F. Tallman, D. Greenblatt & S. Paul, pp. 537–47. Weinheim: Verlag Chemie.

Davis, L.G. & Cohen, R.K. (1980). Identification of an endogenous peptide-ligand for the benzodiazepine receptor. *Biochemical & Biophysical Research Communication*, **92**, 141–8.

Davis, L.G., Manning, R.W. & Dawson, W.E. (1984). Putative endogenous ligands to the benzodiazepine receptor: what can they tell us? *Drug Development Research*, **4**, 31–7.

de Blas, A.L., Sangameswaran, L., Haney, S.A., Park, D., Abraham, C.J. & Rayner, C.A. (1985). Monoclonal antibodies to benzodiazepines. *Journal of Neurochemistry*, **45**, 1748–53.

De Blasi, A., Cotecchia, S., Mennini, T. (1982). Selective changes of receptor binding in brain regions of aged rats. *Life Sciences*, **31**, 335–40.

Donovan, B.T. (1985) *Hormones and human behaviour. The scientific basis of psychiatry*, Vol. 2. Cambridge University Press.

Dorow, R., Horowski, R., Paschelke, G., Amin, M. & Braestrup, C. (1983). Severe anxiety induced by FG 7142, a β-carboline ligand for benzodiazepine receptors. *The Lancet*, **ii**, 98–9.

Duka, T., Höllt, V. & Herz, A. (1979). In vivo receptor occupation by benzodiazepines and correlation with the pharmacological effect. *Brain Research*, **179**, 147–56.

Eder, U., Neef, G., Huth, A., Rahtz, D., Schmiechen, R., Braestrup, C.T., Nielsen, M., Christensen, J.A., Engelstoft, M. & Schou, H. (1981). Beta-carboline-3-carboxylate acid derivatives useful as psychotherapeutic agents. *European Patent* no. 0 030 254.

Ehlert, F.J., Roeske, W.R., Gee, K.W. & Yamamura, H.I. (1983). An allosteric model for benzodiazepine receptor function. *Biochemical Pharmacology*, **32**, 2375–83.

Ehrin, E., Johnström, P., Stone-Elander, S. & Nilsson, L.G. (1984). Preparation and preliminary positron emission tomography studies of ^{11}C-Ro 15–1788, a selective benzodiazepine receptor antagonist. *Acta Pharmaceutica Suecica*, **21**, 183–8.

Emrich, H.M. & Lund, R. (1985). Effect of the benzodiazepine antagonist Ro 15–1788 on sleep after sleep withdrawal. *Pharmacopsychiatry*, **18**, 171–3.

Emrich, H.M., Sonderegger, B. & Mai, N. (1984). Action of the benzodiazepine antagonist Ro 15–1788 in humans after sleep withdrawal. *Neuroscience Letters*, **47**, 369–73.

Enna, S.J. (1984). Receptor regulation. In *Receptors in the nervous system, Handbook of neurochemistry* (2nd edn), ed. A. Lajtha, pp. 629–38, New York: Raven Press.

Essman, E.J. & Valzelli, L. (1981). Brain benzodiazepine receptor changes in the isolated aggressive mouse. *Pharmacological Research Communication*, **13**, 665–71.

Fehske, K.J. & Müller, W.E. (1982). β-Carboline inhibition of benzodiazepine receptor binding in vivo. *Brain Research*, **238**, 286–91.

Fehske, K.J., Müller, W.E., Platt, K.L. & Stillbauer, A.E. (1981). Inhibition of benzodiazepine receptor binding by several tryptophan and indole derivatives. *Biochemical Pharmacology*, **21**, 3016–19.

Fehske, K.J., Zube, I., Borbe, H.O., Wollert, U. & Müller, W.E. (1982). β-Carboline binding indicates the presence of benzodiazepine receptor subclasses in the bovine central nervous system. *Naunyn-Schmiedeberg's Archives of Pharmacology*, **319**, 172–7.

Fernholm, B., Nielsen, M. & Braestrup, C. (1979). Absence of brain specific benzodiazepine receptors in cyclostomes and elasmobranchs. *Comparative Biochemistry and Physiology*, **620**, 209–11.

Ferrero, P., Guidotti, A., Conti-Tronconi, B. & Costa, E. (1984). A brain octadecaneuropeptide generated by tryptic digestion of DBI (diazepam binding inhibitor) functions as a proconflict ligand of benzodiazepine recognition sites. *Neuropharmacology*, **23**, 1359–62.

Fields, H.L. & Levine, J.D. (1984). Placebo analgesia: a role for endorphins? *Trends in Neurosciences*, **8**, 271–3.

File, S.E. (1984). Behavioural pharmacology of benzodiazepines. *Progress in Neuro-psychopharmacology & Biological Psychiatry*, **8**, 19–31.

File, S.E., Green, A.R., Nutt, D.J. & Vincent, N.D. (1984). On the convulsant action of

Ro 5–4864 and the existence of a micromolar benzodiazepine binding site in rat brain. *Psychopharmacology*, **82**, 199–202.

File, S.E., Lister, R.G. & Nutt, D.J., (1982). The anxiogenic action of benzodiazepine antagonists. *Neuropharmacology*, **21**, 1033–7.

File, S.E. & Pellow, S. (1985). The effects of PK 11195, a ligand for benzodiazepine binding sites, in animal tests of anxiety and stress. *Pharmacology, Biochemistry & Behavior*, **23**, 737–41.

File, S.E. & Pellow, S. (1986). Intrinsic actions of the benzodiazepine receptor antagonist Ro 15–1788. *Psychopharmacology*, **88**, 1–11.

File, S.E., Pellow, S. & Jensen, L.H. (1986). Actions of the β-carboline ZK 93 426 in an animal test of anxiety and the holeboard; interaction with Ro 15–1788. *Journal of Neural Transmission*, **65**, 103–14.

Fisch, H.U., Baktir, G., Karlaganis, G. & Bircher, J. (1986). Excessive effects of benzodiazepines in patients with cirrhosis of the liver: a pharmacodynamic or a pharmacokinetic problem? *Pharmacopsychiatry*, **19**, 14.

Fisher, T.E., Davis, L.G., Tuchek, J.M., Johnson, D.D. & Crawford, R.D. (1985). Benzodiazepine receptors and seizure susceptibility in epileptic fowl. *Canadian Journal of Physiology and Pharmacology*, **63**, 85–8.

Fishman, M.C. (1979). Endogenous digitalis-like activity in mammalian brain. *Proceedings of the National Academy of Sciences, USA*, **76**, 4661–3.

Fride, E., Dan, Y., Gavish, M. & Weinstock, M. (1985). Prenatal stress impairs maternal behavior in a conflict situation and reduces hippocampal benzodiazepine receptors. *Life Sciences*, **36**, 2103–9.

Fuxe, K. & Agnati, L.F. (1985). Receptor–receptor interactions in the central nervous system. A new integrative mechanism in synapses. *Medical Research Reviews*, 5, 441–82.

Fuxe, K., Agnatil, L.F., Bolme, P., Höfkelt, T., Lidbrink, P., Ljungdahl, A., Perez de la Mora, M. & Ögren, S.O. (1975). The possible involvement of GABA mechanisms in the action of benzodiazepines on central catecholamine neurons. In *Mechanism of action of benzodiazepine*, ed. E. Costa & P. Greengard, pp. 45–62. New York: Raven Press.

Gaillard, J.-M. & Blois, R. (1983). Effect of the benzodiazepine antagonist Ro 15–1788 on flunitrazepam induced sleep changes. *British Journal of Clinical Pharmacology*, **15**, 529–36.

Gallager, D.W., Lakoski, J.M., Gonsalves, S.F. & Rauch, S.L. (1984). Chronic benzodiazepine treatment decreases postsynaptic GABA sensitivity. *Nature*, **308**, 74–5.

Gath, U., Weidenfeld, J., Collins, G.I. & Hadad, H. (1984). Electrophysiological aspects of benzodiazepine antagonists Ro 15–1788 and Ro 15–3505. *British Journal of Clinical Pharmacology*, **18**, 541–7.

Gentsch, C., Lichtsteiner, M. & Feer, H. (1981). ^{3}H-Diazepam binding sites in roman high- and low-avoidance rats. *Experientia*, **37**, 1315–16.

Goetz, C., Bourgoin, S., Cesselin, F., Brandi, A., Bression, D., Martinet, M., Peillon, F. & Hamon, M. (1983). Alterations in central neurotransmitter receptor binding sites following estradiol implantation in female rats. *Neurochemistry International*, 5, 375–83.

Gonsalves, S.F. & Gallager, D.W. (1985). Spontaneous and Ro 15–1788 induced reversal of subsensitivity to GABA following chronic benzodiazepines. *European Journal of Pharmacology*, **110**, 163–70.

Goodman, L.S. & Gilman, A. (1970). *The pharmacological basis of therapeutics* (4th ed). New York: Macmillan Publishing Co.

Goodman, L.S. & Gilman, A. (1980) *The pharmacological basis of therapeutics* (6th ed). New York: Macmillan Publishing Co.

Grandison, L., Cavagnini, F., Schmid, R., Invitta, S.C. & Guidotti, A. (1982). GABA and benzodiazepine binding sites in human anterior pituitary tissue. *Journal of Clinical Endocrinology & Metabolism*, **54**, 597–601.

Gray, J.A. (1971). Sex differences in emotional behaviour in mammals including man. Endocrine bases. *Acta Psychologica*, **35**, 29–46.

Greenblatt, D.J. & Shader, R.I. (1978). Dependence, tolerance, and addiction to benzodiazepines: clinical and pharmacological considerations. *Drug Metabolism Reviews*, **8**, 13–28.

Grimm, V.E. & Hershkowitz, N. (1981). The effect of chronic diazepam treatment on discrimination performance and ^{3}H-flunitrazepam binding in the brains of shocked and nonshocked rats. *Psychopharmacology*, **74**, 132–6.

Guidotti, A., Forchetti, C.M., Corda, M.G., Konkel, D., Bennett, C.D. & Costa, E. (1983). Isolation, characterization, and purification to homogeneity of an endogenous polypeptide with agonistic action on benzodiazepine receptors. *Proceedings of the National Academy of Sciences, USA*, **80**, 3531–5.

Guzman, F., Cain, M., Larscheid, P., Hagen, T., Cook, J.M., Schweri, M., Skolnik, P. & Paul, S.M. (1984). Biomimetic approach to potential benzodiazepine receptor agonists and antagonists. *Journal of Medicinal Chemistry*, **27**, 564–70.

Haefely, W.E. (1980). Biological basis of the therapeutic effects of benzodiazepines. In *Benzodiazepines today and tomorrow*, ed. R.G. Priest, U.V. Filho, R. Amrein & M. Skreta, pp. 19–45. Lancaster: MTP Press.

Haefely, W. (1983). Antagonists of benzodiazepines: functional aspects. In *Benzodiazepine recognition site ligands: biochemistry and pharmacology*, ed. G. Biggio & E. Costa, pp. 73–93. New York: Raven Press.

Haefely, W. (1984*a*). Actions and interactions of benzodiazepine agonists and antagonists at GABAergic synapses. In *Actions and interactions of GABA and benzodiazepines*, ed. N.G. Bowery, pp. 263–85. New York: Raven Press.

Haefely, W. (1984*b*). Pharmacological profile of two benzodiazepine partial agonists: Ro 16–6028 and Ro 17–1812. *Clinical Neuropharmacology*, **7**, 670–1.

Haefely, W. (1985). Tranquilizers. In *Psychopharmacology 2, Part 1: Preclinical psychopharmacology*, ed. D.G. Grahame-Smith, pp. 92–182. Amsterdam: Elsevier Science Publishers.

Haefely, W., Kulcsar, A., Möhler, H., Pieri, L., Polc, P. & Schaffner, R. (1975). Possible involvement of GABA in the central actions of benzodiazepines. In *Mechanism of action of benzodiazepines*, ed. E. Costa & P. Greengard, pp. 131–52. New York: Raven Press.

Haefely, W., Kyburz, E., Gerecke, M. & Möhler, H. (1985). Recent advances in the molecular pharmacology of benzodiazepine receptors and in the structure–activity relationships of their agonists and antagonists. *Advances in Drug Research*, **14**, 165–322.

Haefely, W., Pieri, L., Polc, P. & Schaffner, R. (1981). General pharmacology and neuropharmacology of benzodiazepine derivatives. In *Handbook of experimental pharmacology*, vol. 55/II, ed. F. Hoffmeister & G. Stille, pp. 13–262. Berlin: Springer Verlag.

Haefely, W., Polc, P., Pieri, L., Schaffner, R. & Laurent, J.-P. (1983). Neuropharmacology of benzodiazepines: synaptic mechanisms and neural basis of action. In *The benzodiazepines from molecular biology to clinical practice*, ed. E. Costa, pp. 21–66. New York: Raven Press.

Halperin, J., Schaeffer, R., Galvez, L. & Malave, S. (1983). Ouabain-like activity in human cerebrospinal fluid. *Proceedings of the National Academy of Sciences, USA*, **80**, 6101–4.

Hamon, M. & Soubré, P. (1983). Searching for endogenous ligand(s) of central benzodiazepine receptors. *Neurochemistry International*, **6**, 663–72.

Hanbauer, I. & Sanna, E. (1986). Endogenous modulator for nitrendipine binding sites. *Clinical Neuropharmacology*, **9**, suppl. 4, 220–2.

Hantraye, P., Kaijima, M., Prenant, C., Guibert, B., Sastre, J., Crouzel, M., Naquet, R., Comar, D. & Maziere, M. (1984). Central type benzodiazepine binding sites: a positron emission tomography study in the baboon's brain. *Neuroscience Letters*, **48**, 115–20.

Häring, P., Stähli, C., Schoch, P., Takacs, B., Staehelin, T. & Möhler, H. (1985). Monoclonal antibodies reveal structural homogeneity of γ-aminobutyric acid/benzodiazepine receptors in different brain areas. *Proceedings of the National Academy of Sciences USA*, **82**, 4837–41.

Hattori, H., Ito, M. & Mikawa, H. (1985). γ-Aminobutyric acid, benzodiazepine binding sites and γ-aminobutyric acid concentrations in epileptic EL mouse brain. *European Journal of Pharmacology*, **119**, 217–23.

Hirsch, J.D., Garrett, K.M. & Beer, B. (1985). Heterogeneity of benzodiazepine binding sites: a review of recent research. *Pharmacology, Biochemistry & Behavior*, **23**, 681–5.

Höfkelt, T., Johannson, O., Ljungdahl, A., Lundberg, J.M. & Schultzberg, M. (1980). Peptidergic neurones. *Nature*, **284**, 515–21.

Holck, M. & Osterrieder, W. (1985). The peripheral high affinity benzodiazepine binding site is not coupled to the cardiac Ca^{2+} channel. *European Journal of Pharmacology*, **118**, 293–301.

Horton, R.W., Prestwich, S.A. & Meldrum, B.S. (1982). γ-Aminobutyric acid and benzodiazepine binding sites in audiogenic seizure-susceptible mice. *Journal of Neurochemistry*, **39**, 864-70.

Hunkeler, W., Möhler, H., Pieri, L., Polc, P., Bonetti, E.P., Cumin, R., Schaffner, R. & Haefely, W. (1981). Selective antagonists of benzodiazepines. *Nature*, **290**, 514–16.

Hunt, P., Husson, J.-M. & Raynaud, J.-P. (1979). A radioreceptor assay for benzodiazepines. *Journal of Pharmacy and Pharmacology*, **31**, 448–51.

Insel, T.R., Ninan, P.T., Aloi, J., Jimerson, D.C., Skolnick, P. & Paul, S.M. (1984). A benzodiazepine receptor-mediated model of anxiety. *Archives of General Psychiatry*, **41**, 741–50.

Jacqmin, P. & Lesne, M. (1984). Comparison between radio-immunoassay and radio-receptor-assay for the measurement of benzodiazepines in biological samples. *Journal de Pharmacie Belge*, **39**, 5–14.

Jensen, L.H., Petersen, E.N., Braestrup, C., Honoré, T., Kehr, W., Stephens, D.N., Schneider, H., Seidelmann, D. & Schmiechen, R. (1984). Evaluation of the β-carboline ZK 426 as a benzodiazepine receptor antagonist. *Psychopharmacology*, **83**, 249–56.

Jochemsen, R., van Rijn, P.A., Hazelzet, T.G.M. & Breimer, D.D. (1983). Assay of midazolam and brotizolam in plasma by a gas chromatographic and a radioreceptor technique. *Pharmaceutisch Weekblad Scientific Edition*, **5**, 308–12.

Johansen, J., Taft, W.C., Yang, J., Kleinhaus, A.L. & DeLorenzo, R.J. (1985). Inhibition of Ca^{2+} conductance in identified leach neurons by benzodiazepines. *Proceedings of the National Academy of Sciences, USA*, **82**, 3935–9.

Johnson, D.A.W. (1983). Benzodiazepines in depression. In *Benzodiazepines divided*, ed. M.R. Trimble, pp. 247–59. Chichester: John Wiley & Sons.

Johnston, G.A.R. & Skerritt, J.H. (1984). GABArins and the nexus between GABA and benzodiazepine receptors. In *Actions and interactions of GABA and benzodiazepines*, ed. N.G. Bowery, pp. 179–89. New York: Raven Press.

Kalaria, R.N. & Prince, A.K. (1986). Decreased neurotransmitter receptor binding in striatum and cortex from adult hypothyroid rats. *Brain Research*, **364**, 268–74.

Karobath, M. (1983). Critique: Endogenous ligand(s) of benzodiazepine receptors? *Neurochemistry International*, **6**, 673–4.

Kataoka, Y., Gutman, Y., Guidotti, A., Panula, P., Wroblewski, J., Cosenza-Murphy, D., Wu, J.Y. & Costa, E. (1984). Intrinsic GABAergic system of adrenal chromaffin cells. *Proceedings of the National Academy of Sciences, USA*, **81**, 3218–22.

Kish, St J., Fox, I.H., Kapur, B.M., Lloyd, K., Hornykiewicz, O. (1985*a*). Brain benzodiazepine receptor binding and purine concentration in Lesch–Nyhan syndrome. *Brain Research*, **336**, 117–23.

Kish, St J., Perry, T.L. & Hornykiewicz, O. (1984). Benzodiazepine receptor binding in cerebellar cortex: observations in olivopontocerebellar atrophy. *Journal of Neurochemistry*, **42**, 466–9.

Kish, St J., Perry, T.L., Sweeney, V.P. & Hornykiewicz, O. (1985*b*). Brain γ-aminobutyric acid and benzodiazepine receptor binding in dialysis encephalopathy. *Neuroscience Letters*, **58**, 241–4.

Kish, St J., Shannak, K.S., Perry, T.L. & Hornykiewicz, O. (1983). Neuronal [^{3}H]benzodiazepine binding and levels of GABA, glutamate, and taurine are normal in Huntington's disease cerebellum. *Journal of Neurochemistry*, **41**, 1495–7.

Kley, H., Scheidemantel, U., Bering, B. & Müller, W.E. (1983). Reverse stereoselectivity of opiate and benzodiazepine receptors for the opioid benzodiazepine tifluadom. *European Journal of Pharmacology*, **87**, 503–4.

Klotz, U. (1984). Clinical pharmacology of benzodiazepines. *Progress in Clinical Biochemistry and Medicine*, **1**, 117–67.

Klotz, U., Ziegler, G. & Reimann, I.W. (1984). Pharmacokinetics of the selective benzodiazepine antagonist Ro 15–1788 in man. *European Journal of Clinical Pharmacology*, **27**, 115–17.

Korneyev, A.Y. & Factor, M.I. (1981). Increase of benzodiazepine binding to the membranes isolated in the presence of diazepam. *European Journal of Pharmacology*, **71**, 127–40.

Kraepelin, E. (1892). *Über die Beeinflussung einfacher psychischer Vorgänge durch einige Arzneimittel*. p. 227. Jena: Gustav Fischer Verlag.

Kraus, V.M.B., Dasheiff, R.M., Fanelli, R.J. & McNamara, J.O. (1983). Benzodiazepine receptor declines in hippocampal formation following limbic seizures. *Brain Research*, **277**, 305–9.

Krespan, B., Springfiled, S.A., Haas, H. & Geller, H.M. (1984). Electrophysiological studies on benzodiazepine antagonists. *Brain Research*, **295**, 265–74.

Kuhar, M.J. (1983). Radiohistochemical localization of benzodiazepine receptors. In *Pharmacology of benzodiazepines* ed. E. Usdin, P. Skolnick, J.F. Tallman Jr., D. Greenblatt & St M. Paul, pp. 149–54. Weinheim: Verlag Chemie.

Kuhn, W., Neuser, D. & Przuntek, H. (1981). [^{3}H]Diazepam displacing activity in human cerebrospinal fluid. *Journal of Neurochemistry*, **37**, 1045–7.

Lader, M. (1978). Benzodiazepines, the opium of the masses? *Neuroscience*, **3**, 159–65.

Lader, M.H. & Davies, H.C. (1986). *Drug treatment of neurotic disorders. Focus on alprazolam*. Edinburgh: Churchill Livingstone.

Laduron, P.M. (1984). Criteria for receptor sites in binding studies. *Biochemical Pharmacology*, **33**, 833–9.

Lal, H. & Harris, C. (1985). Interoceptive stimuli produced by an anxiogenic drug are mimicked by benzodiazepine antagonists in rats pretreated with isoniazid. *Neuropharmacology*, **7**, 677–9.

Lal, H., Mann, P.A. Jr., Shearman, G.T. & Lippa, A.S. (1981). Effect of acute and chronic pentylenetetrazol treatment on benzodiazepine and cholinergic receptor binding in rat brain. *European Journal of Pharmacology*, **75**, 115–19.

Lamb, R.J. & Griffiths, R.R. (1985). Effects of repeated Ro 15–1788 administration in benzodiazepine-dependent baboons. *European Journal of Pharmacology*, **110**, 257–61.

Langer, S.Z., Raisman, R. Tahraoui, L., Scatton, B., Niddam, R. Lee, C.R. & Claustre, Y. (1984). Substituted tetrahydro-β-carbolines are possible candidates as endogenous ligand of the [^{3}H]imipramine recognition site. *European Journal of Pharmacology*, **98**, 153–4.

Lapin, I.P. (1981). Non-specific, non-selective and mild increase in the latency of pentylenetrazol seizures produced by large doses of the putative endogenous ligands of the benzodiazepine receptor. *Neuropharmacology*, **20**, 781–6.

Lapin, I.P. (1983). Structure–activity relationships in kynurenine, diazepam and some putative endogenous ligands of the benzodiazepine receptors. *Neuroscience & Biobehavioral Reviews*, **7**, 107–18.

Lascelles, P.T. (1983). Clinical laboratory aspects of therapeutic monitoring for benzodiazepines. In *Benzodiazepines divided*, ed. M.R. Trimble, pp. 209–27: Chichester: John Wiley & Sons.

Laux, G. (1982). Einteilungs- und Differenzierungsmöglichkeiten der Benzodiazepine. *Fortschritte der Medizin*, **100**, 2179–86.

Lichtstein, D., Minc, D., Bourrit, A., Deutsch, J., Karlish, S.J.D., Belmaker, H., Rimon, R. & Palo, J. (1985). Evidence of the presence of 'ouabain like' compounds in human cerebrospinal fluid. *Brain Research*, **325**, 13–19.

Lippa, A.S., Coupet, J., Greenblatt, E.N., Klepner, C.A. & Beer, B. (1979). A synthetic non-benzodiazepine ligand for benzodiazepine receptors: a probe for investigating neuronal substrates of anxiety. *Pharmacology, Biochemistry & Behavior*, **11**, 99–106.

Lippa, A.S., Sano, M.C., Coupet, J., Klepner, C.A. & Beer, B. (1978). Evidence that benzodiazepine receptors reside on cerebellar Purkinje cells: studies with 'nervous' mutant mice. *Life Sciences*, **23**, 2213–18.

Lippke, K.P., Müller, W.E. & Schunack, W.G. (1985). β-Carbolines as benzodiazepine receptor ligands. 2. Synthesis and benzodiazepine receptor affinity of β-carboline-3-carboxylic acid amides. *Journal of Pharmaceutical Sciences*, **74**, 676–80.

Lippke, K.P., Müller, W.E. & Schunack, W. (1987). Oligopeptide der β-Carbolin-3-carbonsäure – Synthese und Affinität zu Benzodiazepinrezeptoren. *Archive der Pharmazie (Weinheim)*, **320**, 145–53.

Lippke, K.P., Schunak, W., Wenning, W. & Müller, W.E. (1983). β-Carbolines as benzodiazepine receptor ligands: 1. Synthesis and benzodiazepine receptor interaction of esters of β-carboline-3-carboxylic acid. *Journal of Medicinal Chemistry*, **26**, 499–503.

Lowenstein, P.R., Rosenstein, R., Caputti, E. & Cardinali, D.P. (1984). Benzodiazepine binding sites in human pineal gland. *European Journal of Pharmacology*, **106**, 399–403.

Lukas, S.E. & Griffiths, R.R. (1982). Precipitated withdrawal by a benzodiazepine receptor antagonist (Ro 15–1788) after 5 days of diazepam. *Science*, **217**, 1161–3.

MacDonald, J.F., Barker, J.L., Paul, St M., Marangos, P.J. & Skolnick, P. (1979). Inosine may be an endogenous ligand for benzodiazepine receptors on cultured spinal neurons. *Science*, **205**, 715–17.

Mackerer, C.R., Kochman, R.L., Bierschank, B.A. & Bremner, S.S. (1978). The binding of [^{3}H]diazepam to rat brain homogenates. *The Journal of Pharmacology & Experimental Therapeutics*, **206**, 405–13.

McNamara, J.O., Peper, A.M. & Patrone, V. (1980). Repeated seizures induce long-term increase in hippocampal benzodiazepine receptors. *Proceedings of the National Academy of Sciences, USA*, **77**, 3029–32.

McNicholas, L.F., Martin, W.R. & Pruitt, T.A. (1985). N-Desmethyldiazepam physical dependence in dogs. *The Journal of Experimental Pharmacology and Therapeutics*, **235**, 368–76.

Maggi, A., Zucchi, I. & Perez, J. (1984). GABA-receptor and diazepam binding site up-regulation by sex steroid hormones in CNS of rat. *Collegium Internationale Neuro-Psychopharmacologicum 14th congress*. Florence (Italy), abstract F-291.

Maiewsky, S.F., Larscheid, P., Cook, J.M. & Mueller, G.P. (1985). Evidence that a benzodiazepine receptor mechanism regulates the secretion of pituitary β-endorphin in the rat. *Endocrinology*, **117**, 474–80.

Manchon, M., Kopp, N., Bobillier, P. & Miachon, S. (1985). Autoradiographic and quantitative study of benzodiazepine binding sites in human hippocampus. *Neuroscience Letters*, **62**, 25–30.

Mantione, C.R., Weissman, B.A., Goldman, M.E., Paul, S.M. & Skolnick, P. (1984). Endogenous inhibitors of 4′-^{3}H-chlordiazepam (Ro 5–4864) binding to 'peripheral' sites for benzodiazepines. *FEBS Letters*, **176**, 68–74.

Marangos, P.J. & Crawley, J.N. (1982). Chronic benzodiazepine treatment increases [^{3}H]muscimol binding in mouse brain. *Neuropharmacology*, **21**, 81–4.

Marangos, P.J., Patel, J., Hirata, F., Sondheim, D., Paul, S.M., Skolnick, P. & Goodwin, F.K. (1981*a*). Inhibition of diazepam binding by tryptophan derivates including melatonin and its brain metabolite n-acetyl-5-methoxy kynurenamine. *Life Sciences*, **29**, 259–67.

Marangos, P.J., Patel, J., Skolnick, P. & Paul, S.M. (1983). Endogenous 'benzodiazepine-like' agents. In *Pharmacology of benzodiazepines*, ed. E. Usdin, P. Skolnick, J.F. Tallman, D. Greenblatt & S. Paul, pp. 519–27. Weinheim: Verlag Chemie.

Marangos, P.J., Trams, E., Clark-Rosenberg, R.L., Paul, S.M. & Skolnick, P. (1981*b*). Anticonvulsant doses of inosine result in brain levels sufficient to inhibit [^{3}H]diazepam binding. *Psychopharmacology*, **75**, 175–8.

Martin, I.L., Brown, C.L. & Doble, A. (1983). Multiple benzodiazepine receptors: structures in the brain or structures in the mind? A critical review. *Life Sciences*, **32**, 1925–33.

Matsumoto, K., Saito, K.I. & Fukuda, H. (1983). Centrally specific and GABA-insensitive inhibition of benzodiazepine binding by prostaglandins (A_1, A_2 and B_2). *Journal of Pharmacolino-dynamics*, **6**, 784–6.

Mazière, M., Godot, J.M., Berger, G., Baron, J.C., Comar, D., Cepeda, C., Menini, C. & Naquet, R. (1981). Positron tomography. A new method for in vivo brain studies of benzodiazepine, in animal and man. In *GABA and benzodiazepine receptors*, ed. E. Costa, pp. 273–86. New York: Raven Press.

Medina, J.H. & De Robertis, E. (1985). Benzodiazepine receptor and thyroid hormones: in vivo and in vitro modulation. *Journal of Neurochemistry*, **44**, 1340–4.

Medina, J.H., Novas, M.L. & De Robertis, E. (1983*a*). Changes in benzodiazepine receptors by acute stress: Different effects of chronic diazepam or Ro 15–1788 treatment. *European Journal of Pharmacology*, **96**, 181–5.

Medina, J.H., Novas, M.L., Wolfman, C.N.V., Levi de Stein, M. & De Robertis, E. (1983*b*). Benzodiazepine receptors in rat cerebral cortex and hippocampus undergo rapid and reversible changes after acute stress. *Neurosciences*, **9**, 331–5.

Mele, L., Sagratella, S. & Massotti, M. (1984). Chronic administration of diazepam in rats causes changes in EEG patterns and in coupling between GABA receptors and benzodiazepine binding sites in vitro. *Brain Research*, **323**, 93–102.

Memo, M., Spano, P.F. & Trabucchi, M. (1981). Brain benzodiazepine receptor changes during ageing. *Journal of Pharmacy & Pharmacology*, **33**, 64.

Mennini, T. & Garattini, S. (1983). Benzodiazepine receptor binding in vivo: pharmakokinetic and pharmacological significance. In *Benzodiazepine recognition site ligands: biochemistry and pharmacology*, ed. G. Biggio & E. Costa, pp. 189–99. New York: Raven Press.

Merz, W.A. (1984). Partial benzodiazepine agonists: initial results in man. *Clinical Neuropharmacology*, **7**, 672–3.

Mestre, M., Carriot, T., Belin, C., Uzan, A., Renault, C., Dubroeucq, M.C., Gueremy, C., Doble, A. & Le Fur, G. (1984). Electrophysiological and pharmacological evidence that peripheral type benzodiazepine receptors are coupled to calcium channels in the heart. *Life Sciences*, **36**, 391–400.

Mestre, M., Carriot, T., Belin, C., Uzan, A., Renault, C., Dubroeucq, M.C., Guérémy, C. & Le Fur, G. (1985). Electrophysiological and pharmacological characterization of peripheral benzodiazepine receptors in a guinea pig heart preparation. *Life Sciences*, **35**, 953–62.

Mintrun, M.A., Raichle, M.E., Kilbourn, M.R., Wooten, G.F. & Welch, M.J. (1984). A quantitative model for the in vivo assessment of drug binding sites with positron emission tomography. *Annals of Neurology*, **15**, 217–27.

Mizoule, J., Gauthier, A., Uzan, A., Renault, C., Dubroeucq, M.C., Guérémy, C. & Le Fur, G. (1985). Opposite effects of two ligands for peripheral type benzodiazepine binding sites, PK 11195 and Ro 5–4864, in a conflict situation in the rat. *Life Sciences*, **36**, 1059–68.

Möhler, H. (1981). Benzodiazepine receptors: are there endogenous ligands in the brain? *Trends in Pharmacological Sciences*, **2**, 116–19.

Möhler, H. & Okada, T. (1977). Benzodiazepine receptor: demonstration in the central nervous system. *Science*, **198**, 849–51.

Möhler, H. & Okada, T. (1978). The benzodiazepine receptor in normal and pathological human brain. *The British Journal of Psychiatry*, **133**, 261–8.

Möhler, H., Okada, T. & Enna, S.J. (1978). Benzodiazepine and neurotransmitter receptor binding in rat brain after chronic administration of diazepam or phenobarbital. *Brain Research*, **156**, 391–5.

Möhler, H., Polc, P., Cumin, R., Pieri, L. & Kettler, R. (1979). Nicotinamide is a brain constituent with benzodiazepine-like actions. *Nature*, **278**, 563–5.

Möhler, H. & Richards, J.G. (1983). Benzodiazepine receptors in the central nervous system. In *The benzodiazepines from molecular biology to clinical practice*, ed. E. Costa, pp. 93–116. New York: Raven Press.

Moingeon, P., Bidart, J.M., Alberici, G.F. & Bohuon, C. (1983). Characterization of a peripheral-type benzodiazepine binding site on human circulating lymphocytes. *European Journal of Pharmacology*, **92**, 147–9.

Montaldo, A., Serra, M., Concas, A., Corda, M.G., Mele, S. & Biggio, G. (1984). Evidence for the presence of benzodiazepine receptor subclasses in different areas of the human brain. *Neuroscience Letters*, **52**, 263–8.

Morgan, P.F. & Stone, T.W. (1983). Actions of 6-aminonicotinamide on benzodiazepine receptors in rat CNS. *Neuroscience Letters*, **40**, 51–4.

Morin, A.M. (1984). β-carboline kindling of the benzodiazepine receptor. *Brain Research*, **321**, 151–4.

Morin, A.M., Tanaka, I.A. & Wasterlain, C.G. (1981). Norharman inhibition of ^{3}H-diazepam binding in mouse brain. *Life Sciences*, **28**, 2257–63.

Morin, A.M., Watson, A.L. & Wasterlain, C.G. (1983). Kindling of seizures with norharman, a β-carboline ligand of benzodiazepine receptors. *European Journal of Pharmacology*, **88**, 131–4.

Müller, W.E. (1981*a*). The benzodiazepine receptor. An update. *Pharmacology*, **22**, 153–61.

Müller, W.E. (1981*b*). Der Benzodiazepinrezeptor: Eigenschaften und Bedeutung für Pharmakologie, Psychiatrie und Neurologie. *Medizinische Monatsschrift für Pharmazeuten*, **4**, 174–84.

Müller, W.E. (1982*a*). The benzodiazepine receptor. A summary. In *Neuroreceptors*, ed. H. Hucho, pp. 3–13. Berlin: Walter de Gruyter & Co.

Müller, W.E. (1982*b*). Molekularer Wirkungsmechanismus der Benzodiazepine. *Münchner Medizinische Wochenschrift*, **124**, 879–83.

Müller, W.E. (1985). Benzodiazepine receptor interactions of arfendazam, a novel 1,5-benzodiazepine. *Pharmacopsychiatry*, **18**, 10–11.

Müller, W.E., Fehske, K.J., Borbe, H.O., Wollert, U., Nanz, C. & Rommelspacker, H. (1981). On the neuropharmacology of harmane and other β-carbolines. *Pharmacology, Biochemistry & Behavior*, **14**, 693–9.

Müller, W.E., Fehske, K.J. & Schläfer, S.A.C. (1986*a*). Structure of binding sites on albumin. In *Drug-protein binding*, ed. M.M. Reidenberg & S. Erill, pp. 7–23. New York: Praeger Publishers.

Müller, W.E., Groh, B., Bub, O., Hofmann, H.P. & Kreiskott, H. (1986*b*). In vitro and in vivo studies of the mechanism of action of arfendazam, a novel 1,5-benzodiazepine. *Pharmacopsychiatry*, **19**, 314–15.

Müller, W.E., Rick, S. & Brunner, F. (1986*c*). Drug binding to human α_1-acid glycoprotein. Focus on a single binding site. In *Protein binding and drug transport*, ed. J.P. Tillement & E. Lindenlaub, pp. 29–44. Stuttgart: Schattauer Verlag.

Müller, W.E., Schläfer, U., Wollert, U. (1978*a*). Benzodiazepine receptor binding in rat spinal cord membranes. *Neuroscience Letters*, **9**, 239–43.

Müller, W.E., Schläfer, U., Wollert, U. (1978*b*). Benzodiazepine receptor binding: The interactions of some non-benzodiazepine drugs with specific [^{3}H]diazepam binding to rat brain synaptosomal membranes. *Naunyn-Schmiedeberg's Archives of Pharmacology*, **305**, 23–6.

Müller, W.E. & Stillbauer, A.E. (1983). Benzodiazepine hypnotics: time course and potency of benzodiazepine receptor occupation after oral application. *Pharmacology, Biochemistry & Behavior*, **18**, 545–9.

Müller, W.E. & Wollert, U. (1973). Characterization of the binding of benzodiazepines to human serum albumin. *Naunyn-Schmiedeberg's Archives of Pharmacology*, **280**, 229–37.

Müller, W.E. & Wollert, U. (1975). Benzodiazepines: Specific competitors for the binding of L-tryptophan to human serum albumin. *Naunyn-Schmiedeberg's Archives of Pharmacology*, **288**, 17–27.

Müller, W.E. & Wollert, U. (1979). Human serum albumin as a silent receptor for drugs and endogenous substances. *Pharmacology*, **19**, 59–67.

Müller-Oerlinghausen, B. (1986). Prescription and misuse of benzodiazepines in the Federal Republic of Germany. *Pharmacopsychiatry*, **19**, 8–13.

Murphy, K.M.M., Gould, R.J., Largent, L. & Snyder, S.H. (1983). A unitary mechanism of calcium antagonist drug action. *Proceedings of the National Academy of Sciences, USA*, **80**, 860–4.

Nagy, A. & Lajtha, A. (1983). Thyroid hormones and derivatives inhibit flunitrazepam binding. *Journal of Neurochemistry*, **40**, 414–17.

Niehoff, D.L. & Whitehouse, P.J. (1983). Multiple benzodiazepine receptors autoradiographic localization in normal human amygdala. *Brain Research*, **276**, 237–45.

Nielsen, M. Braestrup, C. & Squires, R.F. (1978). Evidence for a late evolutionary appearance of brain-specific benzodiazepine receptors: an investigation of 18 vertebrate and 5 invertebrate species. *Brain Research*, **141**, 342–6.

Niznik, H.B., Burnham, W.M. & Kish, S.J. (1984). Benzodiazepine receptor binding following amygdala-kindled convulsions: Differing results in washed and unwashed brain membranes. *Journal of Neurochemistry*, **43**, 1732–6.

Niznik, H.B., Kish, S.J. & Burnham, W.M. (1983). Decreased benzodiazepine receptor binding in amygdala-kindled rat brain. *Life Sciences*, 5, 425–30.

Nunn, D.J., Robertson, H.A. & Peterson, M.R. (1983). Elevated benzodiazepine receptor density in forebrain of the mutant mouse 'trembler'. *Experimental Neurology*, **82**, 245–7.

Nutt, D. (1983). Pharmacological and behavioural studies of benzodiazepine antagonists and contragonists. In *Benzodiazepine recognition site ligands: biochemistry and pharmacology*, ed. G. Biggio & E. Costa, pp. 153–73. New York: Raven Press.

Nutt, D.J. & Minchin, M.C.W. (1983). Studies on [^{3}H]diazepam and [^{3}H]ethyl-β-carboline carboxylate binding to rat brain in vivo. II. Effects of electroconvulsive shock. *Journal of Neurochemistry*, **41**, 1513–17.

Oakley, N.R., Jones, B.J. & Straughan, D.W. (1984). The benzodiazepine receptor ligand CL 218.872 has both anxiolytic and sedative properties in rodents. *Neuropharmacology*, **23**, 797–802.

Olsen, R.W. (1981). The GABA postsynaptic membrane receptor-ionophore complex site of action of convulsant and anticonvulsant drugs. *Molecular & Cellular Biochemistry*, **39**, 261–79.

Olsen, R.W. (1982). Drug interactions at the GABA receptor-ionophore complex. *Annual Review of Pharmacology & Toxicology*, **22**, 245–77.

Olsen, R.W., Wamsley, J.K., Mccabe, R.T., Lee, R.J. & Lomax, P. (1985). Benzodiazepine/γ-aminobutyric acid receptor deficit in the midbrain of the seizure-susceptible gerbil. *Proceedings of the National Academy of Sciences, USA*, **82**, 6701–5.

Ongini, E. & Barnett, A. (1984). Hypnotic specificity of benzodiazepines. *Clinical Neuropharmacology*, **7**, 812–13.

Overstreet, D.H. & Yamamura, H.I. (1979). Receptor alteration and drug tolerance. *Life Sciences*, **25**, 1865–78.

Owen, F., Cross, A.J., Crow, T.J., Lofthouse, R. & Poulter, M. (1981). Neurotransmitter receptors in brain in schizophrenia. *Acta Psychiatrica Scandinavica*, **63**, supp. 291, 20–7.

Owen, F., Lofthouse, R. & Bourne, R.C. (1979). A radioreceptor assay for diazepam and its metabolites in serum. *Clinica Chimica Acta*, **93**, 305–10.

Owen, F., Poulter, M., Waddington, J.L., Mashal, R.D. & Crow, T.J. (1983). [^{3}H]Ro 5–4864 and [^{3}H]flunitrazepam binding in kainate-lesioned rat striatum and in temporal cortex of brains from patients with senile dementia of the Alzheimer type. *Brain Research*, **278**, 373–5.

Patel, J.B., Stengel, J., Malick, J.B. & Enna, S.J. (1984). Neurochemical characteristics of rats distinguished as benzodiazepine responders and non-responders in a new conflict test. *Life Sciences*, **34**, 2647–53.

Paul, St M. & Skolnick, P. (1978). Rapid changes in brain benzodiazepine receptors after experimental seizures. *Science*, **202**, 892–4.

Paul, St M., Syapin, P.J., Paugh, B.A., Moncada, V. & Skolnick, P. (1979). Correlation between benzodiazepine receptor occupation and anticonvulsant effects of diazepam. *Nature*, **281**, 688–9.

Pedigo, N.W., Schoemaker, H., Morelli, M., McDougal, J.N., Malick, J.B., Burks, T.F. & Yamamura, H.I. (1981). Benzodiazepine receptor binding in young, mature and senescent rat brain and kidney. *Neurobiology of Aging*, **2**, 83–8.

Pellow, S. (1985). Can drug effects on anxiety and convulsions be separated? *Neuroscience & Biobehavioral Reviews*, **9**, 55–73.

Pellow, S. & File, S.E. (1984). Characteristics of an atypical benzodiazepine, Ro 5–4864. *Neuroscience & Behavioral Reviews*, **8**, 405–13.

Penney, J.B., Jr. & Young, A.B. (1982). Quantitative autoradiography of neurotransmitter receptors in Huntington disease. *Neurology*, **32**, 1391–5.

Perret, G. & Simon, P. (1984). Le radiorécepteur essai: Principles et applications à la pharmacologie. *Journal de Pharmacologie (Paris)*, **15**, 265–86.

Persson, A., Erling, E., Eriksson, L., Farde, L., Hedström, C.G., Litton, J.E., Mindus, P. & Sedvall, G. (1985). Imaging of ^{11}C-labelled Ro 15–1788 binding to benzodiazepine receptors in the human brain by positron emission tomography. *Journal of Psychiatric Research*, **19**, 609–22.

Petersen, E.N., Jensen, L.H., Drejer, L.H. & Honoré, T. (1986). New perspectives in benzodiazepine receptor pharmacology. *Pharmacopsychiatry*, **19**, 4–6.

Petersen, E.N. & Lassen, J.B. (1981). A water lick conflict paradigm using drug experienced rats. *Psychopharmacology*, **75**, 236–9.

Phelps, M.E. & Mazziotta, J.C. (1985). Positron emission tomography: human brain function and biochemistry. *Science*, **228**, 799–809.

Placheta, P. & Karobath, M. (1979). Regional distribution of Na^+-independent GABA and benzodiazepine binding sites in rat CNS. *Brain Research*, **178**, 550–83.

Polc, P., Laurent, J.P., Scherschlicht, R. & Haefely, W. (1981). Electrophysiological studies on the specific benzodiazepine antagonist Ro 15–1788. *Naunyn-Schmiedeberg's Archives of Pharmacology*, **316**, 317–25.

Porceddu, M.L., Corda, M.G., Sanna, E. & Biggio, G. (1985). Increase in nigral type 2 benzodiazepine recognition sites following striatonigral denervation. *European Journal of Pharmacology*, **112**, 265–7.

Prezioso, P.J. & Neale, J.H. (1983). Benzodiazepine receptor binding by membranes from brain cell cultures following chronic treatment with diazepam. *Brain Research*, **288**, 354–8.

Reeves, P.M. & Schweizer, M.P. (1983). Aging, diazepam exposure and benzodiazepine receptors in rat cortex. *Brain Research*, **270**, 376–9.

Regan, J.W., Roeske, W.R. & Yamamura, H.I. (1980). The benzodiazepine receptor: Its development and its modulation by α-aminobutyric acid. *The Journal of Pharmacology & Experimental Therapeutics*, **212**, 137–43.

Rehavi, M., Ventura, I. & Sarne, Y. (1984). Demonstration of endogenous 'imipramine like' material in rat brain. *Life Sciences*, **36**, 687–93.

Reisine, T.D., Overstreet, D., Gale, K., Rossor, M., Iversen, L. & Yamamura, H.I. (1980*a*). Benzodiazepine receptors: the effect of GABA on their characteristics in human brain and their alteration in Huntington's disease. *Brain Research*, **199**, 79–88.

Reisine, T.D., Rossor, M., Spokes, E., Iversen, L.L. & Yamamura, H.I. (1980*b*). Opiate and neuroleptic receptor alterations in human schizophrenic brain tissue. In *Receptors* *for neurotransmitters and peptide hormones*, ed. G. Pepeu, M.J. Kuhar & S.J. Enna, pp. 443–50. New York: Raven Press.

Reisine, T.D., Wastek, G.J., Speth, R.C., Bird, E.D. & Yamamura, H.I. (1979). Alterations in the benzodiazepine receptor of Huntington's diseased human brain. *Brain Research*, **165**, 183–7.

Rickels, K. (1981). Benzodiazepines: use and misuse. In *Anxiety: new research and changing concepts*, ed. D.F. Klein & J. Rabkin, pp. 1–12. New York: Raven Press.

Roberts, E. (1984). γ-Aminobutyric acid (GABA): from discovery to visualization of GABAergic neurons in the vertebrate nervous systems. In *Actions and interactions of GABA and benzodiazepines*, ed. N.G. Bowery, pp. 1–25. New York: Raven Press.

Robertson, H.A. (1979). Benzodiazepine receptors in emotional and non-emotional mice: comparison of four strains. *European Journal of Pharmacology*, **56**, 163–6.

Robertson, H.A. (1980). Audiogenic seizures: increased benzodiazepine receptor binding in a susceptible strain of mice. *European Journal of Pharmacology*, **66**, 249–52.

Robertson, H.A., Martin, I.L. & Candy, J.M. (1978). Differences in benzodiazepine receptor binding in maudsley reactive and maudsley non-reactive rats. *European Journal of Pharmacology*, **50**, 455–7.

Rodgers, R.J. & Waters, A.J. (1985). Benzodiazepines and their antagonists: a pharmacoethological analysis with particular reference to effects on 'aggression'. *Neuroscience & Biobehavioural Reviews*, **9**, 21–35.

Roemer, D., Buescher, H.H., Hill, R.C., Maurer, R., Petcher, T.J., Zeugner, H., Benson, W., Finner, E., Milkowski, W. & Thies, P.W. (1982). An opioid benzodiazepine. *Nature*, **298**, 759–60.

Rommelspacher, H. (1981). The β-carbolines (Harmanes) – A new class of endogenous compounds: their relevance for the pathogenesis and treatment of psychiatric and neurological diseases. *Pharmacopsychiatria*, **14**, 117–25.

Rommelspacher, H., Brüning, G., Schulze, G. & Hill, R. (1982). The in vivo occurring β-carbolines induce a conflict-augmenting effect which is antagonized by diazepam: correlation to receptor binding studies. In *Neuroreceptors*, ed. H. Hucho, pp. 27–41. Berlin: Walter de Gruyter & Co.

Rommelspacher, H., Damm, H., Strauss, S. & Schmidt, G. (1984). Ethanol induces an increase of harmane in the brain and urine of rats. *Naunyn-Schmiedeberg's Archives of Pharmacology*, **327**, 107–13.

Rommelspacher, H., Nanz, C., Borbe, H.O., Fehske, K.J., Müller, W.E. & Wollert, U. (1980). 1-methyl-β-carboline (harmane), a potent endogenous inhibitor of benzodiazepine receptor binding. *Naunyn-Schmiedeberg's Archives of Pharmacology*, **314**, 97–100.

Rommelspacher, H., Nanz, C., Borbe, H.O., Fehske, K.J., Müller, W.E. & Wollert, U. (1981). Benzodiazepine antagonism by harmane and other β-carbolines in vitro and in vivo. *European Journal of Pharmacology*, **70**, 409–16.

Rosenberg, H.C. & Chiu, T.H. (1981). Regional specificity of benzodiazepine receptor down-regulation during chronic treatment of rats with flurazepam. *Neuroscience Letters*, **24**, 49–52.

Rosenberg, H.C. & Chiu, T.H. (1982*a*). An antagonist-induced benzodiazepine abstinence syndrome. *European Journal of Pharmacology*, **81**, 153–7.

Rosenberg, H.C. & Chiu, T.H. (1982*b*). Nature of functional tolerance produced by chronic flurazepam treatment in the cat. *European Journal of Pharmacology*, **81**, 357–65.

Rote Liste (1986). Aulendorf (Württ.): Editio Cantor Verlag.

Rothe, T., Schliebs, R. & Bigl, V. (1985). Benzodiazepine receptors in the visual structures of monoculary deprived rats. Effect of light and dark adaption. *Brain Research*, **329**, 143–50.

Ruff, M.R., Pert, C.B., Weber, R.J., Wahl, L.M., Wahl, S.M. & Paul, S.M. (1985). Benzodiazepine receptor-mediated chemotaxis of human monocytes. *Science*, **229**, 1281–3.

Ruhland, M., Liepmann, H. & Muesch, H.R. (1985). 1,2-Anellated 1,4-benzodiazepine derivatives – a new class of antipsychotics. *Pharmacopsychiatry*, **18**, 174–7.

Saletu, B., Grünberger, J., Linzmayer, L. & Sieghart, W. (1984). Zur zentralen Wirkung hoher Benzodiazepindosen: Quantitative Pharmako-EEG- und psychometrische Studien mit Prazepam. In *Forschungen zur Biologischen Psychiatrie*, ed. A. Hopf & H. Beckmann, pp. 271–94. Berlin: Springer-Verlag.

Samson, Y., Hantraye, P., Baron, J.C., Soussalinde, F., Comar, D. & Mazière, M. (1985). Kinetics and displacement of ^{11}C Ro 15–1788, a benzodiazepine antagonist, studied in human brain in vivo by positron tomography. *European Journal of Pharmacology*, **110**, 247–51.

Sandler, M. (1982). The emergence of tribulin. *Trends in Pharmacological Sciences*, **3**, 471–2.

Sandler, M. (1983). Benzodiazepines: Studies on a possible endogenous ligand. In *Benzodiazepines divided*, ed. M.R. Trimble, pp. 139–47. Chichester: John Wiley & Sons.

Sandler, M., Glover, V., Clow, A. & Armando, I. (1983). Endogenous benzodiazepine receptor ligand – monoamine oxidase inhibitor activity in urine. In *Pharmacology of benzodiazepines*, ed. E. Usdin, P. Skolnick, J.F. Tallman, D. Greenblatt & S. Paul, pp. 583–9. Weinheim: Verlag Chemie.

Sangameswaran, L. & de Blas, A.L. (1985). Demonstration of benzodiazepine-like molecules in the mammalian brain with a monoclonal antibody to benzodiazepines. *Proceedings of the National Academy of Sciences, USA*, **82**, 5560–4.

Sauer, G., Wille, W. & Müller, W.E. (1984). Binding studies in the Lurcher mutant suggest an uneven distribution of putative benzodiazepine receptor subclasses in the mouse cerebellum. *Neuroscience Letters*, **48**, 333–8.

Scatchard, G. (1949). The attractions of proteins for small molecules and ions. *Annals of the New York Academy of Sciences*, **51**, 660-72.

Schafer, D.F., Fowler, J.M., Munson, P.J., Thakur, A.K., Waggoner, J.G. & Jones, E.A. (1983). Gamma-aminobutyric acid and benzodiazepine receptor binding in an animal model of fulminant hepatic failure. *Journal of Laboratory & Clinical Medicine*, **102**, 870–80.

Schallek, W., Horst, W.D. & Schlosser, W. (1979). Mechanisms of action of benzodiazepines. *Advances in Pharmacology & Chemotherapy*, **16**, 45–87.

Schatzberg, A.F., Altesman, R.I. & Cole, J.O. (1983). An update of the use of benzodiazepines in depressed patients. In *Pharmacology of benzodiazepines*, ed. E. Usdin, P. Skolnick, J.F. Tallman, D. Greenblatt & S.M. Paul, pp. 45–51. Weinheim: Verlag Chemie.

Scherkl. R. & Frey, H.H. (1986). Physical dependence on clonazepam in dogs. *Pharmacology*, **32**, 18–24.

Schoch, P., Häring, P., Takacs, B., Stähli, C. & Möhler, H. (1984). A GABA/benzodiazepine receptor complex from bovine brain: purification, reconstitution and immunological characterization. *Journal of Receptor Research*, **4**, 189–200.

Schoch, P., Richards, J.G., Häring, P., Takacs, B., Stähli, C., Staehelin, T., Haefely, W. & Möhler, H. (1985). Co-localization of $GABA_A$ receptors and benzodiazepine receptors in the brain shown by monoclonal antibodies. *Nature*, **314**, 168–171.

Schoemaker, H., Morelli, M., Deshmukh, P. & Yamamura, H.I. (1982). [^{3}H]Ro 5–4864 benzodiazepine binding in the kainate lesioned striatum and Huntington's diseased basal ganglia. *Brain Research*, **248**, 396–401.

Schöpf, J. (1983). Withdrawal phenomena after long-term administration of benzodiazepines, a review of recent investigations. *Pharmacopsychiatry*, **16**, 1–8.

Schöpf, J., Laurian, S., Le, P.K. & Gaillard, J.-M. (1984). Intrinsic activity of the benzodiazepine antagonist Ro 15–1788 in Man: an electrophysiological investigation. *Pharmacopsychiatry*, **17**, 79–83.

Schweitzer, J.W., Bonnet, K.A. & Friedhoff, A.J. (1984). Receptor adaptation to psychotropic drugs. In *Receptors in the nervous system, Handbook of neurochemistry* (2nd edn), vol. 6, ed. A. Lajtha, pp. 639–60. New York: Raven Press.

Scollo-Lavizzari, G. (1983). First clinical investigation of the benzodiazepine antagonist Ro 15–1788 in comatose patients. *European Neurology*, **22**, 7–11.

Scollo-Lavizzari, G. (1984). The anticonvulsant effect of the benzodiazepine antagonist Ro 15–1788: an EEG study in 4 cases. *European Neurology*, **23**, 1–6.

Scollo-Lavizzari, G. & Matthis, H. (1985). Benzodiazepine antagonist (Ro 15–1788) in ethanol intoxication: a pilot study. *European Neurology*, **24**, 352–4.

Scollo-Lavizzari, G. & Steinmann, E. (1985). Reversal of hepatic coma by benzodiazepine antagonist (Ro 15–1788). *The Lancet*, **i**, 1324.

Sellers, E.M., Naranjo, C.A., Khouw, V. & Greenblatt, D.J. (1983). Binding of benzodiazepines to plasma proteins. In *Pharmacology of benzodiazepines*, ed. E. Usdin, P. Skolnick, J.F. Tallman, D. Greenblatt & S.M. Paul, pp. 271–84. Weinheim: Verlag Chemie.

Shephard, R.A., Jackson, H.F., Broadhurst, P.L. & Deakin, J.P.W. (1984). Relationships between Hyponeophagia, diazepam sensitivity and benzodiazepine receptor binding in eighteen rat genotypes. *Pharmacology, Biochemistry & Behavior*, **20**, 845–84.

Shephard, R.A., Nielsen, E.B. & Broadhurst, P.L. (1982). Sex and strain differences in benzodiazepines receptor binding in Roman rat strains. *European Journal of Pharmacology*, **77**, 327–30.

Sher, P.K. (1983). Reduced benzodiazepine receptor binding in cerebral cortical cultures chronically exposed to diazepam. *Epilepsia*, **24**, 313–20.

Sher, P.K., Study, R.E., Mazzetta, J., Barker, J.L. & Nelson, P.G. (1983). Depression of benzodiazepine binding and diazepam potentiation of GABA-mediated inhibition after chronic exposure of spinal cord cultures to diazepam. *Brain Research*, **268**, 171–6.

Sherwin, A., Matthew, E., Blain, M. & Guevremont, D. (1986). Benzodiazepine receptor binding is not altered in human epileptogenic cortical foci. *Neurology*, **36**, 1380–2.

Shibla, D.B., Gardell, M.A. & Neale, J.H. (1981). The insensitivity of developing benzodiazepine receptors to chronic treatment with diazepam, GABA and muscimol in brain cell cultures. *Brain Research*, **210**, 471–4.

Shibuya, H., Gale, K. & Pert, C.B. (1980). Supersensitivity to GABA's effect on benzodiazepine receptors develops after striatonigral lesions. *European Journal of Pharmacology*, **62**, 243–4.

Shoemaker, D.W., Cummins, J.T., Bidder, T.G., Boettger, H.G. & Evans, M. (1980). Identification of harmane in the rat arcuate nucleus. *Naunyn-Schmiedeberg's Archives of Pharmacology*, **310**, 227–30.

Sieghart, W. (1985). Benzodiazepine receptors: multiple receptors or multiple conformations? *Journal of Neural Transmission*, **63**, 191–208.

Sieghart, W., Eichinger, A., Riederer, P. & Jellinger, K. (1985). Comparison of benzodiazepine receptor binding in membranes from human or rat brain. *Neuropharmacology*, **24**, 751–9.

Sigel, E., Stephenson, F.A., Mamalaki, C. & Barnard, E.A. (1984). The purified GABA/benzodiazepine/barbiturate receptor complex: four types of ligand-binding sites and the interactions between them are preserved in a single isolated protein complex. *Journal of Receptor Research*, **4**, 175–88.

Silverstein, F.S., Johnston, M.V., Hutchinson, R.J. & Edwards, N.L. (1985). Lesch-Nyhan syndrome: CSF neurotransmitter abnormalities. *Neurology*, **35**, 907–11.

Simmonds, M.A. (1984). Physiological and pharmacological characterization of the actions of GABA. In *Actions and interactions of GABA and benzodiazepines*, ed. N.G. Bowery, pp. 27–43. New York: Raven Press.

Skerritt, J.H., Davies, L.P., Chen Chow, S. & Johnston, G.A.P. (1982). Contrasting regulation by GABA of the displacement of benzodiazepine antagonist binding by benzodiazepine agonists and purines. *Neuroscience Letters*, **32**, 169–74.

Skerritt, H.J. & MacDonald, R.L. (1984). Benzodiazepine receptor ligand actions on GABA responses, β-carbolines, purines. *European Journal of Pharmacology*, **101**, 135–41.

Skolnick, P., Hommer, D., Paul, St M. (1983). Benzodiazepine antagonists. In *Pharmacology of benzodiazepines*, ed. E. Usdin, P. Skolnick, J. Tallmann, D. Greenblatt & S. Paul, pp. 441–54. Weinheim: Verlag Chemie.

Skolnick, P., Marangos, P.J., Goodwin, F.K., Edwards, M., Paul, S. (1978*a*). Identification of inosine and hypoxanthine as endogenous inhibitors of [^{3}H]diazepam binding in the central nervous system. *Life Sciences*, **23**, 1473–80.

Skolnick, P., Ninan, P., Insel, T., Crawley, J. & Paul, S. (1984). A novel chemically induced animal model of human anxiety. *Psychopathy*, **17**, suppl. 1, 25–36.

Skolnick, P., Paul, St M. & Marangos, P.J. (1980). Purines as endogenous ligands of the benzodiazepine receptor. *Federation Proceedings*, **39**, 3050–5.

Skolnick, P., Syapin, P.J. & Paugh, B.A. (1978*b*). Reduction in benzodiazepine receptors associated with Purkinje cell degeneration in 'nervous' mutant mice. *Nature*, **277**, 397–8.

Skolnick, P., Syapin, P.J., Paugh, B.A., Moncada, V., Marangos, P.J. & Paul, S.M. (1979). Inosine, an endogenous ligand of the brain benzodiazepine receptor, antagonizes pentylenetetrazole-evoked seizures. *Proceedings of the National Academy of Sciences, USA*, **76**, 1515–18.

Slater, S. & Longman, D.A. (1979). Effects of diazepam and muscimol on GABA-mediated neurotransmission: interactions with inosine and nicotinamide. *Life Sciences*, **25**, 1963–7.

Snodgrass, S.R. (1983). Receptors for amino acid transmitters. In *Handbook of psychopharmacology, 17, Biochemical studies of CNS receptors*, ed. L.L. Iversen, S.S. Iversen & S.H. Snyder, pp. 167–219. New York: Plenum Press.

Snyder, S.H. (1985). Adenosine as a neuromodulator. *Annual Reviews of Neuroscience*, **8**, 103–24.

Sonawane, B.R., Yaffe, S.J. & Shapiro, B.H. (1980). Changes in mouse brain diazepam receptor binding after phenobarbital administration. *Life Sciences*, **27**, 1335–8.

Soubrie, P., Thiebot, M.H., Jobert, A., Montastruc, J.L., Hery, F. & Hamon, M. (1980). Decreased convulsant potency of picrotoxin and pentetrazol and enhanced ^{3}H-flunitrazepam cortical binding following stressful manipulations in rats. *Brain Research*, **189**, 505–17.

Sperk, G. & Schlögl, E. (1979). Reduction of number of benzodiazepine binding sites in the caudate nucleus of the rat after kainic acid injections. *Brain Research*, **170**, 563–7.

Spero, L. (1982). Neurotransmitters and CNS disease: Epilepsy. *The Lancet*, **ii**, 1319–22.

Speth, R.C., Bresolin, N. & Yamamura, H.I. (1979). Acute diazepam administration produces rapid increases in brain benzodiazepine receptor density. *European Journal of Pharmacology*, **59**, 159–60.

Speth, R.C., Johnson, R.W., Regan, J., Reisine, T., Kobayashi, R.M., Bresolin, N., Roeske, W.R. & Yamamura, H.I. (1980). The benzodiazepine receptor of mammalian brain. *Federation Proceedings*, **39**, 3032–8.

Speth, R.C., Wastek, G.J., Johnson, P.C. & Yamamura, H.I. (1978*a*). Benzodiazepine binding in human brain characterization using [^{3}H]flunitrazepam. *Life Sciences*, **22**, 859–66.

Speth, R.C., Wastek, G.J. & Yamamura, H.I. (1978*b*). Benzodiazepine receptors: temperature dependence of [^{3}H]flunitrazepam binding. *Life Sciences*, **24**, 351–8.

Squires, R.F. (1984). Benzodiazepine receptors. In *Handbook of Neurochemistry*, vol. 6, ed. A. Lajtha, pp. 261–306. New York: Plenum Press.

Squires, R.F. & Braestrup, C. (1977). Benzodiazepine receptors in rat brain. *Nature*, **266**, 732–4.

Stephens, D.N., Kehr, W., Wachtel, H. & Schmiechen, R. (1985). The anxiolytic activity of β-carboline derivatives in mice, and its separation from ataxic properties. *Pharmacopsychiatry*, **18**, 167–70.

Sternbach, L.H. (1973). Chemistry of 1,4-benzodiazepines and some aspects of the structure–activity relationship. In *The benzodiazepines*, ed. S. Garrattini, E. Mussini & L.O. Randall, pp. 1–26. New York: Raven Press.

Syapin, P.J. & Rickman, D.W. (1981). Benzodiazepine receptor increase following repeated pentylenetetrazole injections. *European Journal of Pharmacology*, **72**, 117–20.

Tacke, U. & Braestrup, C. (1984). A study on benzodiazepine receptor binding in audiogenic seizure-susceptible rats. *Acta Pharmacologica et Toxicologica*, **55**, 252–9.

Tallman, J.F. & Gallager, D.W. (1985). The GABA-ergic system: a locus of benzodiazepine action. *Annual Reviews of Neuroscience*, **8**, 21–44.

Tallman, J.F., Thomas, J.W. & Gallager, D.W. (1978). GABAergic modulation of benzodiazepine site sensitivity. *Nature*, **274**, 383–5.

Ticku, M.K. (1983). Benzodiazepine–GABA receptor–ionophore complex current concepts. *Neuropharmacology*, **22**, 1459–70.

Tietz, E.I., Rosenberg, H.C. & Chiu, T.H. (1986). Autoradiographic localization of benzodiazepine receptor downregulation. *The Journal of Pharmacology & Experimental Therapeutics*, **236**, 284–92.

Tran, V.T., Snyder, S.H., Major, L.F. & Hawley, R.J. (1980). GABA receptors are increased in brains of alcoholics. *Annals of Neurology*, **9**, 289–92.

Tsang, C.C., Speeg, K.V., Jr. & Wilkinson, G.R. (1982). Aging and benzodiazepine binding in the rat cerebral cortex. *Life Sciences*, **30**, 343–6.

Tyma, J.L., Rosenberg, H.C. & Chiu, T.H. (1984). Radioreceptor assay of benzodiazepines in cerebrospinal fluid during chronic flurazepam treatment in cats. *European Journal of Pharmacology*, **105**, 301–8.

Tyrer, P.F. (1984). Benzodiazepines on trial. *British Medical Journal*, **288**, 1101–2.

Tyrer, P., Owen, R. & Dawling, S. (1983). Gradual withdrawal of diazepam after long-term therapy. *The Lancet*, **i**, 1402–6.

Vaccarino, F.M., Ghetti, B. & Nurnberger, J.I. (1985). Residual benzodiazepine (BZ) binding in the cortex of pcd mutant cerebella and qualitative BZ binding in the deep cerebellar nuclei of control and mutant mice: an autoradiographic study. *Brain Research*, **343**, 70–8.

Vaccarino, F.M., Ghetti, B., Wade, S.E., Rea, M.A. & Aprison, M.H. (1983). Loss of Purkinje cell-associated benzodiazepine receptors spares a high affinity subpopulation: a study with pcd mutant mice. *Journal of Neuroscience Research*, **9**, 311–23.

Voigt, M.M., Davis, L.G. & Wyche, J.H. (1984). Benzodiazepine binding to cultured human pituitary cells. *Journal of Neurochemistry*, **43**, 1106–13.

Waddington, J.L. & Cross, A.J. (1978). Denervation supersensitivity in the striatonigral GABAergic pathway. *Nature*, **276**, 618–20.

Walker, F.O., Young, A.B., Penney, J.B., Dovorini-Zis, K. & Shoulson, I. (1984). Benzodiazepine and GABA receptors in early Huntington's disease. *Neurology*, **34**, 1237–40.

Wang, J.K.T., Taniguchi, T. & Spector, S. (1984). Structural requirements for the binding of benzodiazepines to their peripheral-type sites. *Molecular Pharmacology*, **25**, 349–51.

Watkins, L.R. & Mayer, D.J. (1982). Organization of endogenous opiate and nonopiate pain control systems. *Science*, **216**, 1185–93.

Wauquier, A. & Ashton, D. (1984). The benzodiazepine antagonist, Ro 15–1788, increases REM and slow wave sleep in the dog. *Brain Research*, **308**, 159–61.

White, W.F. & Heller, A.H. (1982). Glycine receptor alteration in the mutant mouse spastic. *Nature*, **298**, 655–7.

Whitehouse, P.J., Muramoto, O., Troncoso, J.C. & Kanazawa, I. (1986). Neurotransmitter receptors in olivopontocerebellar atrophy: an autoradiographic study. *Neurology*, **36**, 193–7.

Wilkinson, M., Bhanot, R., Wilkinson, D.A. & Brawer, J.R. (1983). Prolonged estrogen treatment induces changes in opiate, benzodiazepine and β-adrenergic binding sites in female rat hypothalamus. *Brain Research Bulletin*, **11**, 279–81.

Winokur, A. & Rickels, K. (1984). Withdrawal responses to abrupt discontinuation of desmethyldiazepam. *American Journal of Psychiatry*, **141**, 1427–9.

Woolf, J.H. & Nixon, J.C. (1981). Endogenous effector of the benzodiazepine binding site: purification and characterization. *Biochemistry*, **20**, 4263–9.

Wu, J.-Y., Lin, H.S., Su, Y.Y.T. & Yang, C.Y. (1984). Isolation and purification of benzodiazepine receptor and its endogenous ligand. *Neuropharmacology*, **23**, 881–3.

Wusteman, M., Reynolds, G.P. & Martin, I.L. (1985). Flunitrazepam and muscimol binding to post-mortem brain tissue in epilepsy. *British Journal of Pharmacology*, **85**, 363p.

Yamamura, H.I., Enna, S.J. & Kuhar, M.J. (1978). *Neurotransmitter receptor binding*. New York: Raven Press.

Yokoyama, N., Ritter, B. & Neubert, A.D. (1982). 2-Arylpyrazolo(4,3-c)quinolin-3-ones: novel agonists, partial agonists, and antagonists of benzodiazepines. *Journal of Medicinal Chemistry*, **25**, 337–9.

Young, W.S., III, & Kuhar, M.J. (1979). Autoradiographic localisation of benzodiazepine receptors in the brains of humans and animals. *Nature*, **280**, 393–4.

Ziegler, G., Ludwig, L. & Fritz, G. (1985). Reversal of slow-wave sleep by benzodiazepine antagonist Ro 15–1788. *The Lancet*, **ii**, 510.

Zimmer, G., Ziegler, G., Müller, W.E. & Beckmann, H. (1986). Mögliche intrinsische Aktivität von Ro 15–1788. *Fortschritte der Neurologie und Psychiatrie*, **54**, 18 (Sonderheft).

INDEX